D0790835

GUIDELINE
FROM START
TO FINISH

For Jenny, James and Sophia – R.B.

For Elsevier:

Commissioning Editor: Pauline Graham
Development Editor: Janice Urquhart
Project Manager: Kerrie-Anne Jarvis
Designer: Charles Gray
Illustrator: Richard Morris
Illustration Manager: Merlyn Harvey

HOW TO WRITE A GUIDELINE
FROM START TO FINISH

A HANDBOOK FOR HEALTHCARE PROFESSIONALS

Richard Bowker MA MRCPCH MB BS
Paediatric Specialist Registrar, Nottingham University Hospital NHS Trust,
Nottingham, UK

Monica Lakhanpaul DM MRCP MRCPCH MB BS
Senior Lecturer in Child Health, University of Leicester; Consultant Paediatrician,
Community Child Health Services, Leicester, UK

Maria Atkinson MRCPCH MB ChB
Paediatric Respiratory Specialist Registrar, Nottingham University Hospital
NHS Trust, Nottingham, UK

Kate Armon DM FRCPCH MRCP DCH DRCOG BM BS BMedSc
Consultant Paediatrician, Norfolk and Norwich University Hospitals NHS Trust,
Norwich, UK

Roddy MacFaul FRCP FRCPCH DCH
Consultant Paediatrician, Pinderfields Hospital, Wakefield, UK

Terence Stephenson DM FRCP FRCPCH
Professor of Child Health; Dean, Faculty of Medicine & Health Sciences, Medical
School, University of Nottingham, Nottingham, UK

With a contribution from

Hannah-Rose Douglas BA MSc PhD
Senior Health Economist, National Collaborating Centre for Women and Children's
Health, London, UK

CHURCHILL LIVINGSTONE
ELSEVIER

Edinburgh   London   New York   Oxford   Philadelphia   St Louis Sydney   Toronto 2008

An imprint of Elsevier Limited

First published 2008

ISBN: 978-0-443-10035-2

British Library Cataloguing in Publication Data
A catalogue record for this book is available from the British Library

Library of Congress Cataloging in Publication Data
A catalog record for this book is available from the Library of Congress

Notice
Knowledge and best practice in this field are constantly changing. As new research and experience broaden our knowledge, changes in practice, treatment and drug therapy may become necessary or appropriate. Readers are advised to check the most current information provided (i) on procedures featured or (ii) by the manufacturer of each product to be administered, to verify the recommended dose or formula, the method and duration of administration, and contraindications. It is the responsibility of the practitioner, relying on their own experience and knowledge of the patient, to make diagnoses, to determine dosages and the best treatment for each individual patient, and to take all appropriate safety precautions. To the fullest extent of the law, neither the Publisher nor the Authors assume any liability for any injury and/or damage to persons or property arising out or related to any use of the material contained in this book.

The Publisher

ELSEVIER
your source for books,
journals and multimedia
in the health sciences
www.elsevierhealth.com

Working together to grow
libraries in developing countries

www.elsevier.com | www.bookaid.org | www.sabre.org

ELSEVIER   BOOK AID
                International   Sabre Foundation

The
Publisher's
policy is to use
**paper manufactured
from sustainable forests**

Printed in China

Contents

Preface

Guidelines for healthcare professionals are being developed locally and nationally in an ever increasing number. The quality of these documents varies. A clinical guideline is only useful if it delivers improvements in patient care. A guideline can only deliver benefits for patients if it is used by the healthcare community. The healthcare community are more likely to use a guideline if they see that it is based on the best evidence, it is able to be implemented and they have been involved in the process of its development.

The authors of this book have been involved in national guideline writing for several years. The research conducted and lessons learnt from our experiences have contributed to the current established guideline methodology. We have all had our successes and made our own mistakes.

We have often been asked by our colleagues to write a guideline for their topic of interest, but developing a clinical guideline is a significant undertaking. Previously, to help our colleagues succeed in their projects, we have directed them to the technical manuals of the major guideline institutions. However you cannot learn how to play a sport simply by reading the rule book! Therefore, we have written this book as a practical guide for guideline developers. The book explains the rules of guideline development adding the handy hints and tips we have picked up along the way. We also point out the pitfalls which we have met so others can learn from those who went before.

As the reader begins on their own personal guideline journey, they should be fore warned of the winding roads ahead. But the end result can be very rewarding. By using this book as a guide, hopefully the reader will be able to develop a guideline which delivers improvements in patient care – possibly on a national scale.

R. B.
M. L.
M. A.
K. A.
R. MacF.
T. S.

Acknowledgements

The authors would like to thank the following people: Dr Hannah-Rose Douglas (Senior Health Economist, National Collaborating Centre for Women and Children's Health) for writing Chapter 10: Health economics, which could not even have been started by the other authors; Professor Rhonda Bell (Associate Professor, Alberta Institute for Human Nutrition, University of Alberta, Canada) for her assistance with Chapter 14: Dissemination and implementation; Mr John Tingle (Reader in Health Law, Director of the Centre for Health Law, Nottingham Law School, Nottingham Trent University) for his expertise and suggestions for Chapter 15: Legal issues.

Introduction

Maria Atkinson

Aims

- To define a clinical guideline
- To establish why clinical guidelines are needed
- To provide an overview of guideline development over the last few years
- To explain the terminology used

1

What is a clinical guideline?

Clinical guidelines are often described as *'systematically developed statements to assist practitioner and patient decisions about appropriate health care for specific clinical circumstances'*.[1]

Emphasis should be placed on the words 'assist' and 'appropriate'. Clinical guidelines 'assist', but do not force, specific decisions to be made. 'Appropriate' care is determined by the specific circumstances and by the patient's own views of treatment and risk.

The overall aim of a clinical guideline is to improve patient outcomes.

Guidelines do not constrain practitioners. Guidelines do not produce a culture of 'cook-book medicine'. Guidelines often provoke practitioners to question what they do and why, which is no bad thing. Guidelines are a tool to assist in the art of decision-making. Guidelines are frequently the catalyst to encourage learning about a specific clinical practice.

Guidelines: do we really need them?

As a reader of this book, you are probably contemplating developing a guideline. Therefore, you probably need little persuasion about the value of clinical guidelines. There are, however, many sceptics out there who will.

Example Box 1.1

Mr Bloggs attends your local emergency department with crushing chest pains. His ECG suggests a myocardial infarction.

As healthcare professionals, we may fall into one of three categories when managing a clinical case:
- the novice or rusty practitioner;
- the confident practitioner;
- or the cutting-edge practitioner.

All these types of professional need guidance on how to manage Mr Bloggs, although they may not realize it.

The novice needs basic guidance on what to do.

The confident practitioner needs to be up to date with the best management strategies rather than relying solely on what they did last time.

The cutting-edge practitioner needs to know where the gaps in our knowledge are so that new research can be undertaken according to clinical needs.

Mr Bloggs wants the best available treatment to improve his health outcomes. He doesn't want his health to suffer because his condition struck at a certain time of day or in a certain area of the country.

All these needs can be satisfied with high-quality clinical guidelines.

Note: *Feel free to change this example to one more appropriate to your own field of practice (e.g. the hypertensive patient in your general practice, the patient with gestational diabetes in your antenatal clinic, the depressed patient with suicidal ideation in your outreach service, the patient with a chronic venous ulcer in your community setting, etc.).*

Persuading the sceptics

As you read through this book, you will realize the most important aspect of guideline development is encouraging use of the recommendations by a rather sceptical and conservative population of healthcare professionals. Here are some ways to persuade your colleagues why guidelines are a good thing:

The altruistic view

We all want to do the best for our patients, but how do we know what is the best? When we first qualify we usually rely on what we've been taught. From the time of Hippocrates, teaching medicine has included the passing on of experiences from one generation to another. As individual experiences differ, guidance to peers and students has differed greatly over the years.

The ability to compare experiences improved when medical journals were established several hundred years ago. They provided a forum for discussing clinical practice. However, many such discussions were based on individual, and therefore potentially biased, observations. These observations may not lead to improvements in practice.

In recognition of these biases, rigorous experimental design was defined with the dawning of the randomized controlled trial in the middle of the 20th century. By reducing the bias of the observer successful treatment strategies can be identified with greater confidence. Evidence-based guidelines incorporate the best available evidence into practice recommendations. Therefore, using an evidence-based guideline should hopefully lead to improvements in healthcare standards.

The financial view

Mr Bloggs was treated under the care of a Professor of Cardiology who had just been to a conference on the use of a very expensive monoclonal antibody, which had been used with some benefit in patients with myocardial infarction. Mr Bloggs was treated with this new drug and was discharged home after 3 weeks. Mr Smith, his next door neighbour, was admitted with a similar myocardial infarction and was treated by a different team. He did not receive the new drug but was discharged home after 3 weeks of hospitalization.

- Who received the better treatment?
- Should this new treatment be made available throughout the health service?
- How would this new treatment impact on the rest of the health service budget?

These questions are best answered by looking at the evidence and weighing up the cost-effectiveness for the individual and the health service. Clinical guidelines not only look at the health outcomes of treatments but also look at the health economic outcomes. This is increasingly important when spending in one area of the health service equals reduced spending in another (opportunity costs). Changes in practice which save money without a reduction in health benefits or which cost more but provide better health outcomes should be advocated over those which cost more with little improvement in clinical results.

The litiginous view

Mr Bloggs complained that he did not receive good care in your hospital. In particular, he felt he did not receive the appropriate treatment at the appropriate time. He had a friend who was treated for a similar condition in another hospital and now has much better health than he has. The hospital managers investigate. On asking the staff involved in his care they all say he received the treatments which most patients get in his condition. On asking another team not involved in his care, they say they would have done things quite differently.

The hospital's Patient Claims Department phone their neighbouring hospital and ask them what they do in a similar clinical scenario. This hospital has written down a clinical guideline agreed to by all the staff in the coronary care unit. This has standardized the care within the unit and all staff follow the guidelines if appropriate for that individual patient. When a similar complaint arose at their hospital, they looked back at the care the patient had received and they were satisfied that it was not substandard. The complaint was dropped.

Unfortunately, there were no standards laid down by your hospital for the care of patients with chest pain caused by a myocardial infarction. Even though your hospital felt the care was not substandard, it was concerned about the risk of fighting Mr Bloggs' case. The claim was settled out of court for a 'reasonable' sum. The

3

hospital managers have now identified this as an area of clinical risk. The measures taken to reduce this risk in future include the adoption of a clinical guideline.

Clinical guidelines provide recommendations and standards for the care of patients. They should help reduce risk during clinical episodes. Not only will this reduce the chance of a successful litigation claim, but the hospital insurance scheme may be cheaper every year.

The political view

In the United Kingdom, where health care is provided at a national level by the National Health Service (NHS), there has always been a political will to improve standards of care across the nation. 'A first class service: quality in the new NHS' states: *'All patients in the NHS are entitled to high quality care. This should not depend on the geographic accident of where they happen to live. The unacceptable variations that have grown up in recent years must end. Clinical decisions should be based on the best possible evidence of effectiveness, and all staff should be up to date with the latest developments in their field'.*[2] With this political will came carrots and sticks and statutory obligations.

Healthcare professionals have always been responsible for their actions and the service they provide[3] but they now also have a responsibility to provide evidence of the effectiveness of their practice. The drive to promote best practice and to safeguard standards of care by creating an environment in which excellence in clinical care will flourish has been termed 'clinical governance'.

Clinical governance, though not a new phenomenon, has now become a statutory responsibility for the National Health Service in an attempt to standardize care throughout the country. Its aims are:

- to improve the quality of care provided to patients;
- to make health professionals accountable for their actions;
- and to improve public confidence in their health service by showing them that the 'NHS will not tolerate less than best practice'.[4]

Clinical guidelines are an integral part of clinical governance. They help practitioners to set standards, follow standards, measure standards and ultimately improve standards. They allow Trusts to demonstrate their adoption of best practices. When guidelines are promoted nationally, best practices are adopted throughout the UK, removing the so-called 'postcode lottery' of the NHS. Some of the complex relationships between different groups and processes in clinical governance are represented in Figure 1.1.

Clinical governance players

National Institute of Health and Clinical Excellence

The National Institute of Clinical Excellence began in 1999 as a special health authority in order to reduce variability in clinical decision-making, to improve access to care in the health system and to ensure evidence-based practice within the National Health Service. The remit was extended in 2005 to include health promotion, hence the name change (National Institute of *Health* and Clinical Excellence). It is responsible for encouraging quality improvement by appraising new technologies and drugs, and assessing their clinical and cost effectiveness.

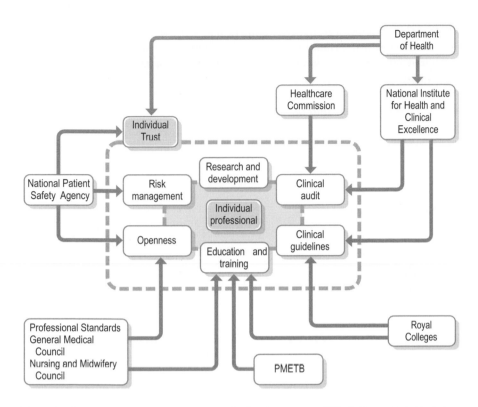

Figure 1.1 Some of the elements and relationships in clinical governance. PMETB, Postgraduate Medical Education and Training Board.

In addition, it is responsible for producing, approving and disseminating clinical guidelines in England and Wales.

Healthcare Commission

The UK government has the responsibility for introducing clinical governance frameworks and for establishing standards which are expected to be met. Other institutions and individuals are responsible for implementing the standards. The standards are monitored by the Healthcare Commission in the UK. This body assesses the performance of Trusts (in both primary care and hospital settings). The audit of guidelines forms a key step in assessing performance.

Individual colleges

The responsible colleges (e.g. Royal College of Nursing, Royal College of Radiologists) set clinical standards and disseminate guidelines via their clinical effectiveness committees. They are also responsible for ensuring the quality of their doctors by developing an appropriate examination structure, encouraging evidence-based practice and having ultimate responsibility for the continuing professional development of their members.

The Hospital Trust or the Primary Health Care Trust

Each Trust chief executive is ultimately responsible for the quality assurance of the Trust. Individual Trusts have developed their own clinical governance plans. They disseminate and implement policies and guidelines developed by the Trust Board and clinical governance committees. They are required to provide evidence to the Healthcare Commission of local activities that promote quality of care for the patients they serve.[2]

Individual directorates and practices

Individual professional groups (e.g. GP practices and hospital directorates) are responsible in their own clinical area for developing and implementing risk management strategies, clinical guidelines, protocols, personal development plans and appraisals, and for the re-validation of their group members.

Individual professionals

Individual health professionals have always been responsible for providing high-quality care to patients. Individuals are accountable to the General Medical Council (GMC) or the Nursing and Midwifery Council (NMC). They are also accountable to individual patients who can sue professionals if they do not consider that they have received care of appropriate quality.[3]

The changing face of guideline development

Guidelines have been produced for many generations and have often been published in the form of personal practice ('this is what I do and it works for me') articles. Then departments started getting together and writing down what they agreed should happen for certain conditions. This exercise was undertaken mainly to give advice to the junior members of their team so that they could work through a problem by themselves.

By the mid 1990s most hospitals in the UK had some form of guidance that they gave in written form to their junior doctors, usually including resuscitation protocols. At the same time professional bodies such as the GMC and the medical and nursing colleges were producing their own statements regarding best practice for a variety of conditions. Other organizations, such as the Resuscitation Council (UK) or the British Thoracic Society, were producing guidelines to be adopted by members of the various colleges.

Suddenly, lots of guidelines were being produced. Anyone with a pen and paper (keyboard and mouse) could write a guideline, but very few were being appraised for their quality. Some guidelines on the same topic, but with different authors, contradicted each other. The reason for the differences arose because of the way guidelines were being developed and the lack of a good appraisal system.

Gobsat

The most common way of producing a national guideline in years gone by has been given the acronym 'GOBSAT' – good old boys sitting around tables. Here a group of (often self-defined) experts would meet and draw up recommendations about their topic of interest. As these professionals had practised in their own individual way for many years without detailed scrutiny of the effectiveness of their treatments, they would often make recommendations which replicated their own practice. This is a very efficient way of writing a guideline but may not lead to effective health improvements.

One improvement to the GOBSAT technique is the introduction of evidence into the round-the-table discussions. However, the majority of the publications used in developing the guidelines were authored by the experts on the panel. Evidence which contradicted the authors' publications would not necessarily be included in the discussions.

The electronic revolution

The next improvement was seen when the use of literature searching software (e.g. MEDLINE) blossomed. Systematic reviews of the literature could be performed to remove bias from the selection of evidence presented to the discussions. The increased publication of meta-analyses and the Cochrane database were highly influential in this aspect. A hierarchy of evidence levels evolved (see Chapter 7), which made recommendation formation a more understandable process.

In the last decade, GOBSAT has been frowned upon and now multidisciplinary panels are used to form recommendations. This way individual biases are diluted. Formal consensus processes (see Chapter 8) are used where evidence is lacking. Larger national organizations have been formed to produce guidelines, such as NICE, the Scottish Intercollegiate Guidelines Network (SIGN) and the New Zealand Guidelines Group (NZGG). These groups are transparent about the way their guidelines are formed, so that any part of the process could be repeated or appraised by others.

Assessment of methodology

Guidelines for guideline developers are now established in Europe. The AGREE (Appraisal of Guidelines REsearch and Evaluation) collaboration has developed a universal appraisal tool which can be applied to any completed guideline to assess how rigorously it has been developed. Most national guideline developers will use the AGREE tool during development to ensure the end product is given the seal of approval. Throughout this book we will be referring to the AGREE collaboration standards so that they can be followed or used in your own guideline development process.

Implementation strategies

Guideline development is a pointless exercise if no-one is going to use or even read the guidelines. Implementation of guidelines is a key part of the development process but has in the past been somewhat neglected. As healthcare professionals are conservative, changing their practice is not easy, especially when it is a change to using someone else's guideline. Part of the reason for formalizing guideline development was to improve user uptake of the evidence-based advice.

High-quality guidelines now include representatives from multiple disciplines and allow all the users of the developing guideline to participate in its formation from an

Table 1.1

Definitions	
Evidence-based medicine	'Evidence based clinical practice is an approach to decision making in which the clinician uses the best evidence available, in consultation with the patient, to decide upon the option which suits that patient best'.[5]
Clinical guideline	Clinical guidelines are recommendations designed to support the decision-making processes in patient care.
Evidence-based guideline	Systematically developed statements to assist practitioner and patient decisions about appropriate health care for specific clinical circumstances. The systematic approach to the inclusion of evidence in the guideline differs from the approach taken by a 'best practice guideline'.
Best practice guideline	Recommendations developed for patient care without the systematic approach used for developing an evidence-based guideline.
Protocol	A protocol is a set of instructions on how to manage a situation. The instructions are expected to be followed in all cases. The difference between a guideline and a protocol is that a guideline helps with decision-making while a protocol should require no judgements to be made. For example, a guideline may recommend a starting dose of insulin in a diabetic patient, whereas a protocol explains the steps required to set up an insulin infusion.
Policy	A policy is a guiding principle designed to influence decisions, actions, etc. For example, it may be policy to follow evidence-based guidelines in your department.
Recommendation	This is the practice statement which the reader of the guideline can follow. It should be easy to understand and implement.
Grade of recommendation	A scoring system has been devised to identify which statements are based on the strongest evidence and which statements are based on the weakest evidence.
Good practice point	A recommendation that will never be subjected to a clinical trial but is obviously sensible practice. For example, it is good practice to keep medical notes (no trial data available!).
Formal consensus process	Where no experimental evidence exists, groups of individuals can make recommendations based on their experiences. A formal approach may produce recommendations which are more likely to be implemented than those produced by a small group of experts (see Chapter 8).
Guideline development group (GDG)	A multidisciplinary panel involved in the decision-making process of recommendation formation. They have the final responsibility for the guideline. The size of the group should be limited to allow for efficient committee meetings (somewhere between 10 and 20 members).
Stakeholder group	A representative body of a group of professionals, who will be affected by the guideline. Due to the limitation in the size of the guideline development group, not all stakeholder groups can be represented on the GDG. Stakeholder groups should have the ability to contribute their members' view to the GDG and be involved in the process from the beginning.

8

Table 1.1

Continued

Systematic search	Evidence searching has been thorough with transparent methodology to try to collect as many relevant sources of information as possible. It will involve an electronic search of more than one database, a hand-search and sometimes contacting individual authors for more data.
Evidence appraisal	Individual papers which are found are subjected to a rigorous and standardized critique, which determines whether they meet the pre-determined standard for inclusion and how their results affect recommendation formation.
Evidence table	A summarized version of individual papers that have been appraised and included for analysis by the guideline development group. They contain an explanation of the type of study, methods and results, and also comments on the strengths and weaknesses of individual studies.
Evidence level	Objective systems have developed to reduce the bias in evidence appraisal. The hierarchies of evidence are based on what type of study is being appraised and whether there are any methodological flaws in the paper. Different systems have been developed (see Chapter 7).
Systematic review	A systematic review attempts to answer a specific question by performing a systematic search of the literature on that topic and appraising the available evidence found. A summary of all the available evidence can be reported in a number of ways depending on the study types and the clinical question asked.
Meta-analysis	This is a specific type of systematic review, where the data from the sources of evidence can be analysed together statistically. Thus, data from multiple small studies can be pooled and analysed as one large study, which may improve the confidence in the findings of the smaller studies and look at results of important subgroups.
Prospective study	A study where the subjects are recruited and followed up over a period to record events as they happen.
Retrospective study	A study where the subjects are identified after specific events have happened, and their previous experiences researched to determine what may have led to the specific event.
Randomized controlled trial	A study to test a specific intervention by randomly allocating two groups of individuals to two different treatments. Randomization reduces selection bias, ensuring that the demographics and disease states of the two groups at recruitment are similar and confounding factors are equally spread across the two groups. Therefore any differences in the treatment outcomes should be down to the intervention not to inherent differences in the two groups.
Cohort study	An observational study which takes a group of individuals sharing a common characteristic (e.g. a disease) and follows them up over time. Prognostic features of the specific subgroups may be identified, and reported as risk factors or protective factors for a worse or better prognosis.

Table 1.1

Continued	
Case–control study	A study which identifies a group of individuals with a common characteristic (cases) and then looks for another group of individuals without that characteristic (controls). All the individuals have their past life events scrutinized to determine which factors differ in the case group compared to the control group, thereby highlighting risk factors for developing the disease. Clearly the controls should be matched as closely as possible to the cases for age, sex and social class, but as no randomization occurs unidentified confounding factors within the populations may cause misinterpretation of any prognostic factors reported.
Case series	A report of several cases of the same disease and the experience of the outcomes. There is no control group.
Diagnostic test study	A study to determine the effectiveness of a test or sign to accurately predict the presence of the specific disease compared to the accuracy of the gold standard test for that disease.
Guideline appraisal	The process by which the guideline methodology and findings are appraised. Most guidelines will be appraised using the AGREE Instrument.[6]
Guideline algorithm	A diagrammatic representation of the recommendations made in the guideline. It demonstrates where key clinical decisions are made and down which treatment path the patient should go.
Care pathway	A tool which can be used as part of the routine clinical documentation to remind staff to follow specific recommendations at specific times in the patient's clinical course.
Guideline technical document	The full-length version of the guideline including which evidence was used to support the recommendations and how the decisions were reached in forming the recommendations. The list of contributors and the stakeholder involvement should be clear as well as methods for dissemination and implementation.
Dissemination	The method of publicizing the document so that it is available for the users of the guideline.
Implementation	The methods employed to get the users to change their practice and use the recommendations developed by the guideline development group.
Audit	The process for setting targets and monitoring performance against agreed standards. An evidence-based guideline is considered to be best clinical practice. An audit of the guideline's use will determine how frequently the guideline recommendations are being followed. Audit should identify both ways of improving performance and also the areas in which the guideline may need to improve.

early stage. By making the process inclusive and transparent it is hoped that doctors, nurses and other allied health professionals can understand the benefits of implementing and using individual guidelines. National guidelines can be implemented at a local level with changes specific for the local requirements. Care pathways (see Chapter 14) are one way of translating guidelines into everyday practice.

However, you plan to implement your guideline, either locally or nationally, enthusiasm and persistence will be required in abundance.

Guideline terminology

Table 1.1 should help to clarify what is meant by the various terms used in guideline development. Unfortunately, these terms have no standard definition and some are used interchangeably. We define in Table 1.1 what is meant by these terms in this book.

Summary

So, do we need clinical guidelines? There will always be those who feel that clinical guidelines remove an individual's ability to practise the art of medicine, and could even stifle progress. Individual experience is a powerful and important aspect of our practice. If guidelines are followed without thought to the individual clinical case, if they have not been written well or if they are out of date, then those who resist the use of guidelines have a very strong argument. However, guidelines will be with us now for as long as clinical governance is practised.

By the end of reading this book, you will be able to find, develop and implement the best quality clinical guidelines, which you will be able to keep updated and will standardize practice within your field. When guidelines are adopted which have been developed with attention to quality and clinical need, the sceptics are left with very little ammunition to fire.

The answer, therefore, to the original question becomes a resounding 'Yes'.
- Guidelines are a necessary part of clinical practice.
- They need to be transparently developed so that users can understand how the recommendations were made.
- Unless a guideline is implemented the whole process will be pointless.

11

References

1. Field MJ, Lohr KN (eds) Clinical practice guidelines: directions for a new program. Institute of Medicine. Washington, DC: National Academy Press, 1990.
2. Secretary of State for Health. A first class service: quality in the new NHS. London: Department of Health, HMSO; 1998.
3. Allen P. Accountability for clinical governance, developing collective responsibility for quality in primary care. BMJ 2000; 321:608–611.
4. Halligan A. Clinical governance, right here, right now. NHS Magazine 2001; 2.
5. Muir Gray JA. Evidence-based healthcare: how to make health policy and management decisions. London: Churchill Livingstone; 1997.
6. The AGREE Collaboration. Appraisal of guidelines for research and evaluation (AGREE Instrument). 2001. www.agreecollaboration.org

Chapter 2

Developing a national guideline

Terence Stephenson

Aims

- To provide an overview for developing a national guideline
- To discuss a timescale for the process

Overview

So you have decided or been commissioned to develop a guideline for national use. For the end product to be taken seriously and implemented it will have to be:

- thoughtfully developed;
- evidence-based;
- transparent.

To produce such a guideline the stages shown in Figure 2.1 need to take place.

Timetable for guideline development

Every evidence-based guideline requires a significant amount of effort and hard work. The minimum amount of time for a comprehensive guideline covering a clinical problem or diagnosis to be completed is probably 18 months but 2 years is more likely.[1] Many of the stages in Figure 2.1 can run concurrently but it is wise to leave plenty of time for each stage to be completed. Be aware that guideline development involves many group discussions, and agreement will take longer than you think. To keep the guideline on track a schedule should be drawn up at the start of the process and you should aim to stick to the deadlines set.

1. Forming a guideline development group

There needs to be a driving force behind the project to keep the momentum going. This driving force comes from the guideline development group and its chair. Selecting group members, inviting them to take part and finding alternatives if initial candidates aren't available will take *6 weeks to 3 months*.

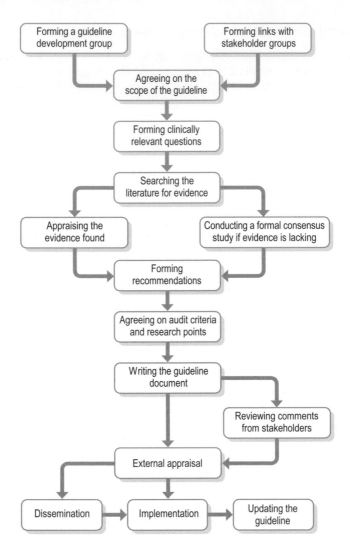

Figure 2.1 The steps involved in producing a national guideline.

2. Forming links with stakeholder groups

The stakeholder groups are identified easily, but finding the right people within each organization who will provide the back-up you require takes multiple letters/emails. Expect to have most of the links established within *3 months*.

3. Agreeing on the scope of the guideline

Where a guideline starts and stops determines the limit of the recommendations. The guideline development group (GDG) will have strong opinions as to what areas they particularly feel the guideline should cover. It will take a GDG meeting to determine this. Therefore it will take at least *1 month*.

4. Forming clinically relevant questions

The scope of the guideline gives the boundaries but the questions will determine the topics the recommendations cover. Again it will take at least one meeting to discuss these issues. The number of questions will impact on the evidence search and appraisal. Most guidelines try to limit the questions but often have more than 20. Time required: *1 to 2 months*.

5. Searching the literature for evidence

Each clinical question will have its own search strategy, so the length of time required to complete this part of the guideline will be determined by the number of questions asked. Each question will take on average 1 day of electronic searching and selecting. However, locating papers may take much longer, especially if interlibrary loans are required which take a couple of weeks to come through. Even NICE don't have electronic access to the British Library medical archives! Time required: *2 to 3 months*.

6. Appraising the evidence found

Again this will depend on how many searches have been performed and how much evidence has been found. Each retrieved paper will take about 2 hours to appraise and summarize into an evidence table. It is mentally exhausting and cannot be done all in one go. Time required: *2 to 3 months*.

7. Conducting a formal consensus study

This is an option which more and more guideline developers, including NICE, are adopting. The timescale will depend on the methodology. If a Delphi consensus process is desired then this will take at least *6 months*.

8. Forming recommendations

Guideline recommendations have to reflect accurately the evidence but also incorporate clinical judgement and health economic arguments. The wording has to be clear so that guideline users are sure about what advice they are being given. The guideline development group has to be satisfied with each recommendation and the discussions can be intense. Each recommendation will often take an hour or so of round table debating in a GDG meeting. The frequency of GDG meetings will be a factor as to how long the finalized recommendations will take to write. Time required: *3 months*.

9. Agreeing on audit criteria and research points

This will take up an hour or so of round table discussions at a GDG meeting if prior email debating has been taking place. Time required: *1 month*.

10. Writing the guideline document

This is dependent on how the workload has been split up. The GDG can be split into topic groups that write individual sections of the guideline. Alternatively, one member can be given the task of putting the whole package together. If good minutes have been taken during each meeting and the evidence tables are ready to 'cut and paste' into an appendix, then the task may not be as arduous as first anticipated. Time required: *2 months*.

11. Reviewing comments from stakeholders

A draft version of the guideline document should be circulated to the stakeholder groups that have been involved during the development phase. Any major problems with the recommendations can be flagged up at this stage before final publication. The GDG will then be in a position to take on board the criticisms and either make adjustments without compromising the evidence-based nature of the recommendations or strengthen the arguments in the document so that the reasoning behind the recommendations is clearer. Time required: *2 months*.

12. External appraisal

This is out of the control of the GDG so it will depend on the workload and method of appraisal undertaken. Time required: *2 to 6 months*.

13. Dissemination and implementation

This is an ongoing process once the guideline is written. Once external appraisal has been completed, it should be possible to disseminate the document in about 2 months by talks, mail-shots and electronic media. Encouraging people to use the guideline may or may not be the responsibility of the GDG but strategies to aid implementation should be discussed during the development process.

14. Updating the guideline

The shelf-life of a guideline is about 3 years. Updating the document requires a meeting of the original GDG. The evidence searches need updating (limited to papers published since the last guideline searches) and feedback from the users of the guideline needs to be incorporated into the updated guideline. Time required: *2 to 3 months*.

There is a lot of work to be organized and delegated. It will be up to individual groups to decide how best to work. It will be near impossible to produce a national guideline with GDG members who are all volunteers for the project. A full-time methodologist or clinical fellow or research nurse is key to providing much of the leg work for the project. Otherwise the guideline will falter, as deadlines are missed due to the group's other work commitments.

Summary

- Keep the process evidence-based and transparent.
- Set aside 2 years for the project.
- Employ a full-time member for the project.

Reference

1. SIGN. Guideline development in 50 easy steps. 2004. www.sign.ac.uk/pdf/50steps.pdf

Chapter 3

Developing local guidelines

Maria Atkinson

Aims

- To discuss the different roles of local and national guidelines
- To provide a framework for developing local guidelines
- To identify useful websites for local guideline development

Evidence-based guidelines take up to 2 years to develop, with a team of dedicated professionals all contributing. These documents need to be revised every 2 to 3 years. Before embarking on such a journey locally, a few questions need to be resolved:

1. How can your department possibly afford to commit scarce resources to write an evidence-based guideline for a small group of practitioners?

2. Why should your department spend time developing its own guideline and another department 5 miles away develop a similar document duplicating the work and spending further precious healthcare resources?

3. How can the guidelines you have developed locally be updated on a regular basis?

The answers to these questions are expanded below, but briefly they are:

1. It can't.

2. It shouldn't if the topic is important enough.

3. Good organization and delegation.

Developing local guidelines compared to national guidelines

Nationally developed guidelines have a number of functions which differ from locally developed guidelines (Table 3.1).

Table 3.1	Some of the key differences between nationally and locally developed guidelines

National guidelines	Local guidelines
Ensure evidence-based practice across the whole healthcare service	Ensure best practice in a local setting
Reduce postcode lottery of patients across geographical borders	Improve standardization of practice by different members of the same team
Have to take into account different patient settings and allow for different healthcare structures nationally to achieve the best clinical goals	Can be very specific about settings and structures within which local practice occurs

Nationally developed guidelines

- National guidelines should ensure that best practice is available to all patients and thus clinical outcomes should not be based on a postcode lottery. Therefore, the recommendations need to be applicable across the whole health service.

- They should champion the translation of expensive research evidence into practice by undertaking a systematic search of all available literature. They should use only expert opinion (consensus) to form recommendations when all searches have found no helpful evidence.

- A wide consultation process needs to take place to ensure that all opinions have been heard before the recommendations are finalized.[1]

- The recommendations need to be implemented at a local level determined by the structures and resources of individual departments.

Locally developed guidelines

- Local guidelines developed from scratch tend to use evidence which is easily available. However, unless a *rigorous* search for evidence has been undertaken and the steps outlined in the rest of this book followed, then the guideline cannot be labelled 'evidence-based'. In other words, local guidelines developed on a shoestring are rarely the all-singing, all-dancing 'evidence-based' guideline and this needs to be acknowledged explicitly.

- The user of the local guideline will be keen to know how things work locally and what preferences their particular department has when managing a clinical condition. Therefore, a local guideline can be based around the practice and consensus of the local experts (e.g. general practitioners with a special interest, hospital consultants, senior nurse practitioners, senior pharmacists).

- The guideline needs to have agreement from all those whose practice will be affected by the guideline recommendations, which may require cross-departmental discussions.

A framework for local guideline formation

The thought of updating or developing a new local guideline fills most of us with dread. This is mainly because the expectations for a local guideline are set too high.

Remember, the guideline is for your team to use. If everyone in your team agrees to the recommendations made and there has been an *open arena* for debate, then that is a perfectly reasonable local guideline.

- However, the team must be aware of 'group think', characterized by the attitudes of President Kennedy's US government prior to the Cuban missile crisis. If everyone starts off thinking the same and every member reinforces the preconceptions of their colleagues, then there is no critical challenge.

- There is consensus – everyone agrees to do the wrong thing!

Developing a new guideline for local use

Search for an evidence-based guideline (see Figure 3.1). Have a look at the sites listed below (see 'Useful websites') to see whether a national guideline already exists. If it does then don't re-invent the wheel!

Also check the relevant websites of the specialty of the guideline you are updating and speak to the lead consultant who may be aware of a guideline in print.

Guideline found

1. Check guideline quality

If you find a guideline the next thing to do is try to decide whether it has been well developed. The most objective way to do this is to use the AGREE tool[2] (see Appendix 1 and Chapter 13).

If it has not been rigorously developed then you should query the validity of the recommendations and consider writing them from scratch.

If it appraises favourably, then move on to the next step.

2. Adapt guideline to local circumstances

Most guidelines need altering to take into account local practice and services. For example, you find a guideline for the management of patients with suspected

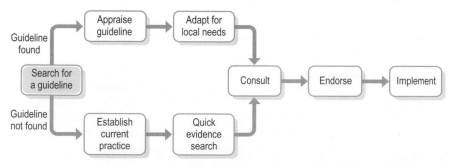

Figure 3.1 Framework for writing new local guidelines.

epilepsy which recommends MRI of the brain for all patients who meet certain criteria. If you work in a hospital which has a CT scanner but no MRI, implementing the guideline will not be straightforward. The guideline will have to be adapted to take into account the local situation and local resources.

3. Consult everyone affected by the guideline

All healthcare professionals work in slightly different ways. If a guideline which is not based on strong evidence recommends the opposite strategy to how someone else has always managed that same problem, they are unlikely to change their practice without some resistance (see Chapter 14). Incorporating their viewpoint in the recommendation and finding the common ground will mean that a guideline is more likely to be implemented.

Changes in practice are never limited to one department. In the epilepsy example above, although the guideline was aimed at the physicians, it will clearly have big repercussions in the Radiology Department.

The earlier a group of individuals is informed of the guideline being developed the more likely they are to participate and contribute. This way potential problems can be ironed out during the development process.

4. Endorse the guideline

There needs to be an official process to say, 'yes, we will use this guideline' or 'no, we won't use this guideline'. There is no point in individuals parachuting a guideline into a department which no-one else has had the option of commenting on. The guideline will be left in limbo, with staff not knowing if it is 'official' or not. See 'Sustainable local guideline development' below for tips on managing a guideline committee, which is a good solution to the endorsing issue.

5. Implement the guideline

See Chapter 14.

Guideline not found

1. Establish current practice

Ask around your colleagues. What do they do when faced with the clinical problem which the guideline covers? Try to present their answers in a flow diagram, following the journey of the patient. Accept that there will be areas where differences in practice exist and highlight these.

This will be the first draft of the guideline.

2. Perform a quick evidence search

Ask your colleagues if they base their practice on any known evidence. If they can give you the references then try to seek these papers out.

If practice is based mainly on experience, check that there is no strong evidence to change practice. Search the following databases for evidence:

The Cochrane Library (for systematic reviews)
(www.thecochranelibrary.com)

DARE – Database of Abstracts of Reviews of Effects (for systematic reviews) (www.thecochranelibrary.com)

Clinical Evidence (for structured evidence-based reviews of topics) (www.clinicalevidence.com)

TRIP – Turning Research Into Practice (for evidence-based reviews of topics) (www.tripdatabase.com)

Bandolier (for appraised evidence within a topic) (www.jr2.ox.ac.uk/bandolier)

N.B. Do not look for primary evidence by performing a MEDLINE search, as this will not count as a systematic literature search and will take you all day to wade through.

Any strong evidence (systematic reviews or randomized controlled trials) found in the four databases above can be used to support your recommendations. If the evidence suggests that your recommendations are not sound then you need to show the evidence to your colleagues and consider re-drafting the guideline. If there is no evidence found then your consensus-based guidelines have much more legitimacy.

Write the recommendations in a way that is easy to understand and easy to access in a hurry. Consider a laminated summary sheet or a 'key points' front page. Excessively long explanations of why the recommendations have been made should be placed in an appendix if they affect the utility of the guideline document.

3. Follow steps 3, 4 and 5 in the section 'Guideline found' above for the rest of the guideline development process.

Updating an existing guideline

1. It's still good practice to go through steps 1–3 above. If you find a good evidence-based guideline you may want to use this in preference to the guideline already in use.

2. If you do not find anything superior to the guideline already in use and there is no new evidence found in the five suggested databases, then it is a case of making sure it is still user-friendly and covers the important points. Discuss with colleagues who have used the guideline, check if there are any gaps where guidance is needed but not provided, or if the advice is confusing. Is the guideline easy to read and use? Check with the front-line end-users (GP partners, SHOs, ward nurses, pharmacists), not the authors or the senior staff who sit on committees but rarely access these documents 'in anger'.

3. Follow steps 3–5 in the section 'Guideline found' to ensure that everyone is happy with and aware of the updated guideline.

At the end of this process you may have:

- a completely new guideline with different recommendations;
- the same guideline but presented in a different format; or
- the same guideline with no changes at all.

Any of these outcomes is acceptable.

- If you are making changes always give every iteration a version number and use the 'track changes' option if using 'Word' with a different font colour to highlight the revisions.
- Make sure the footer contains page numbers and date of revision. (It is extraordinary how often different readers are commenting on different versions and how often revisions are re-revised back to the original text!)

Please also note that many medical guidelines may overlap with nursing guidelines. Please check and liaise with a senior nurse if this is the case. This will ensure that the same advice is being given at all times.

Sustainable local guideline development

Guidelines serve a really useful educational function for all staff, whether in training or fully qualified. They teach staff what to do in specific situations, why they should do it and where the gaps in our knowledge lie. Involving the whole department in guideline development can be a positive step and doesn't need the creation of a new post to fulfil.

1. Endorse

Secondary care

A model which works well for a hospital department is to hold a monthly guideline meeting (instead of a 'Journal club' say) – the guideline committee. Prior to the meeting a draft of a new/updated guideline should be circulated to all interested parties, who are invited to attend. At the meeting there should a brief presentation of the guideline followed by a discussion of key points and any disagreements with the recommendations.

At the end of the process, the guideline should either be:

- endorsed and implemented;
- endorsed with a few changes; or
- rejected with recommendations for the next iteration; a good rule of thumb is not to reject or criticize a colleague's efforts outright without having a thought about what constructive alternative wording or recommendation you would suggest.

Consideration should be given to implementation strategies (see Chapter 14).

Primary care

In primary care, a similar model can be used, although there are likely to be many more national evidence-based guidelines relevant to this more general specialty. Therefore, instead of discussing 'whether' to endorse the new published guideline, the meeting could focus on 'how' to implement them.

2. Update

Guidelines need to be reviewed every 2–3 years. A folder of guidelines in use with 'best before' dates clearly stated should be kept by the guideline committee or on the trust intranet. Individuals should be delegated to update a guideline which is nearing or over its review date and set a deadline for it to be brought to the guideline meeting.

3. Disseminate

Information about guidelines should be given to all new staff at induction – where to find them and how to use them. In hospitals, on every ward round the team can be asked whether the clinical decision followed the guideline or whether there was a valid reason not to. This will encourage further use of the guidelines in everyday practice.

4. Audit

Audit has a key role in the improvement of health services (see Chapter 12). The availability of a guideline which can be audited will help get an audit project started. The process of audit will encourage staff to follow the guideline, as they know they are being 'watched' (the Hawthorne effect).

- This is the thinking underlying inspection of schools and why advanced warning is given rather than snap-shot drop-in teams. The benefit stems from encouraging teams to adopt good practice in advance, not from catching them out in bad practice.

Audit will lead to changes in practice and/or improvements in the guideline as it evolves.

Useful websites

The list below is by no means comprehensive and is merely meant to act as a starting point for those unfamiliar with guideline websites. The list covers only English-language guidelines. However, there are some excellent guidelines and tips on guideline writing contained in many of these sites.

UK

www.library.nhs.uk
National Library for Health: this site contains a guideline finder. Most of the high-quality clinical guidelines are listed here, including those produced by NICE and SIGN, and the site has links to international guidelines.

www.nice.nhs.uk
The National Institute for Health and Clinical Excellence: this site contains all the guidelines which the Department of Health has commissioned for England, Wales and N. Ireland since NICE began in 1998. The guidelines produced by NICE are

the gold standard for nationally developed guidelines, including lots of patient input and health economics.

www.sign.ac.uk
The Scottish Intercollegiate Guidelines Network: this site contains all the guidelines which have been commissioned by NHS Quality Improvement Scotland. Again these are the gold standard for guideline developers but they don't have the health economic input of NICE.

www.cks.library.nhs.uk
Clinical Knowledge Summaries are a Department of Health initiative for primary care guidelines.

ebmg.wiley.com
A collection of evidence-based guidelines for primary care.

Specialty guidelines

www.brit-thoracic.org.uk
The British Thoracic Society publishes national guidelines for the management of respiratory conditions in adults and children.

Royal College websites

Also look through the website of your specialty organization and find out what guidelines they endorse.

International

www.guideline.gov
This is the site of the National Guideline Clearinghouse. This is a US-based site funded by the Department of Health. It has structured abstracts and summaries about guidelines and their development. Links to full-text guidelines, where available, and palm-based downloads.

mdm.ca/cpgsnew/cpgs/index.asp
This is the Canadian Medical Association clinical practice guidelines site.

www.nhmrc.gov.au
This is the site of the Australian Government National Health and Medical Research Council. It has a 'clinical practice guidelines' area which contains several high-quality guidelines.

www.nzgg.org.nz
This is the New Zealand Guidelines Group website. It contains several high-quality guidelines and useful links.

Other

www.agreecollaboration.org
This is the site to locate the AGREE appraisal tool to determine whether the guideline you've found has been rigorously developed.

Summary

- Look for evidence-based guidelines and adapt for local use.
- If developing a new guideline from scratch, keep it simple.
- Developing a means of sustainable local guideline development will provide an excellent training resource.

References

1. Grimshaw J, Eccles M, Russell I. Developing clinically valid guidelines. J Evaluation Clin Practice 1995; 1:37–48.
2. The AGREE Collaboration. Appraisal of guidelines for research and evaluation (AGREE Instrument). 2001. www.agreecollaboration.org

Chapter 4

Getting started – or working back to front

Richard Bowker

Aims

- To describe the process of choosing a guideline topic
- To establish the target audience for the final guideline
- To describe the selection of the guideline development group
- To begin to define the limits of the guideline

Before you begin to put pen to paper, it is important to realize the time and effort which goes into producing an evidence-based guideline. SIGN and NICE take about 18 months to 2 years from start to finish, and they have a number of resources to draw upon which most other guideline developers don't. If you are writing a departmental practice guideline then the process is not as daunting, but it still needs to be documented carefully.

Don't be put off by the journey ahead, merely accept that it will take longer than you think.

Begin at the end

When you start writing a guideline you must bear in mind what will happen to the final document. You may dream of it being accepted nationally, with the clinical course of numerous patients improving, and great acclaim being bestowed upon the authors.

Keep your feet firmly on the ground! Clinical improvements in patient care through using guidelines will be achieved only if the recommendations in the guidelines are sound and they are actually used by clinicians. Clinicians will not use your guideline unless they think the recommendations are sound and relevant to their patients. Demonstrating that the recommendations are 'sound' can be done by using the AGREE Instrument (see below). Proving that clinical improvements have occurred through a guideline will be dealt with in Chapter 12; however, it is often a major challenge.

Table 4.1

Summary of AGREE Instrument guideline assessment tool
Guideline development appraisal
Scope and purpose
Stakeholder involvement
Rigour of development
Clarity and presentation
Applicability
Editorial independence

The AGREE Instrument[1] is the appraisal tool against which your final guideline will be assessed. Go and read this useful document (Appendix 1) before you start developing your guideline (Table 4.1). You will then know the benchmark against which the guideline will be measured.

Document the whole process as you go along referring back to the AGREE Instrument appraisal, so that those who externally assess the guideline will be able to do so easily.

For evidence-based guidelines, the external assessors may be the Royal Colleges or the local guideline committee. Appraisal of the final guideline should be performed externally so that end-users do not need to go through the process individually and they can be confident that the guideline's recommendations are sound.

Secondly, stop thinking about the guideline as 'your' guideline. If it remains 'your' guideline then probably only *you* will read it. Think about including end-users at the beginning, so they too feel they have developed the guideline and will be more inclined to use it.

Topic selection

It is assumed that, having picked up this book, the reader has been asked or is planning to write a guideline on a specific topic. Just take a moment to think about how that topic was chosen. Have there been incidents in clinical practice related to the

Example Box 4.1 Examples of how others choose guideline topics	
NICE	Department of Health and Welsh Assembly identify key topics for guideline development.[2]
SIGN	Any group or individual may propose a guideline topic to SIGN. In addition, SIGN has established specialty subgroups which use established clinical networks to identify a 'wish-list' of guideline topics.[3]
Paediatric accident and emergency research group	A study determined the commonest presenting problems to the emergency department[4] and guidelines for development were decided on the basis of the frequency of these presenting problems and their clinical burden.

28

topic? Are there widely differing practices across the region leading to a 'postcode lottery' of care? Is there uncertainty in a field which needs clarification? Has a new treatment been suggested without agreement of its cost–benefit implications? Is there a need for this guideline at this time or should another topic be considered?

You may not be able to undergo such formal topic selection processes as in Example Box 4.1. At the very least ask your colleagues if they feel there is a need for a guideline on the suggested topic. Record how the topic was selected, as this will be required reading in the 'Scope and Purpose' section of the final guideline documentation (see Appendix 1).

Targeting your audience

Two questions need to be asked:

- Who are the patients in the guideline?
- Who are the professionals using the guideline?

Patient groups

Imagine a patient suffering with the condition related to the guideline topic (e.g. angina). Which patient groups should be included in the guideline?

- All patients suspected of having the condition (e.g. all patients with crushing chest pain radiating down the left arm)
- All patients with a confirmed diagnosis (e.g. symptoms confirmed with exercise EEG)
- All patients referred to hospital (e.g. angina sufferers seen in a cardiology clinic)
- All patients admitted to hospital (e.g. angina sufferers seen acutely in the emergency department or the coronary care unit)

The patient groups which are included will determine where the guideline starts and which health professionals they are likely to encounter.

Professional groups

Two overlapping groups need to be identified: the target users of the guideline and the professionals who may be affected by the guideline being implemented.

1. Who will eventually use the guideline and when?

- Will the guideline be used by all health professionals? Is it specific for nursing staff? Is it specific for a particular grade of doctor? Does it involve more than one discipline at some point?
- Will the guideline be read every time a patient presents with a certain condition? Is it for reference in the middle of the night, so the consultant doesn't have to be woken? When would someone realistically have a chance to pick up the guideline and use it?

29

Example Box 4.2

SIGN guideline (no. 66) 'Diagnosis and management of childhood otitis media in primary care'[5] is relevant for general practitioners (GPs), practice nurses, audiologists, paediatricians, otolaryngologists, audiological physicians, health visitors, social workers, public health physicians, users of services and all other professionals caring for children.

The patient groups included in the guideline are children with suspected acute or chronic otitis media (OM) seen in primary care. This is the largest group of children suffering with OM as most are seen in the community first, and primary care professionals differ in their treatment strategies.

Although the guideline is 'relevant' to all the professionals listed, the target users (i.e. those most likely physically to pick up and read the guideline) are general practitioners and other primary care professionals. The boundaries of the guideline have therefore been set around diagnosis in the community, treatments available in the community and referral criteria for specialist care from the community. The guideline did not make recommendations for specialist treatments of children with otitis media, as that was beyond the scope of the guideline's boundaries.

---

2. Who will be affected by the guideline being implemented?

Imagine the patient's journey through the health system. Who will be involved in their care in some way? All these professional groups will need to be involved in the process of guideline development. For example, the 'Breathing difficulties' guideline[6] (developed by the Paediatric Accident and Emergency Research Group) was developed for the use of senior house officers and gave guidance on who should be investigated with a chest X-ray. Even though radiologists would not be expected to use the guideline in their day to day work, the guidance within it would affect their workload, and so they were given the opportunity and encouraged to contribute.

Thus, by identifying the end-users of the guideline and those affected by the guideline at the beginning you will have identified who will need to be involved in developing the recommendations, where patients will enter the guideline, and will give a rough idea of the boundaries for guideline recommendations. Again, record the patient groups identified ('Scope and Purpose') and the target users identified ('Stakeholder involvement') in the guideline development document.

Selecting a guideline development group and identifying stakeholders

Representation

Guideline development is a group activity. Although a committee-of-one may seem like an efficient way of getting a guideline written, you will find that having the breadth of views and experiences of a group really helps. Even if you are writing a local practice guideline, you still need the final document to be approved by other members of your local team, otherwise it will remain a personal practice guideline. If you are writing a Trust-wide or national guideline, *or* you would like it to be evidence-based, then you need to open the project up to other participants.

A guideline development group (GDG) is a collection of individuals who represent different professional groups' views. Look back at the list of professionals who will be involved in the management of patients relevant to the guideline topic and think how they can be represented on the GDG.

Example Box 4.3

The Paediatric Accident and Emergency Research Group was developing a guideline 'Breathing Difficulty: An evidence based guideline for the management of children presenting with acute breathing difficulty',[6] whose target audience was to be junior doctors in the emergency department/ acute paediatric units, and which could be used for any child whom they encountered with breathing difficulties.

The GDG comprised two paediatric specialist registrars (one of whom was responsible for co-ordinating the guideline), an emergency department consultant, a paediatric emergency department senior nurse, a paediatric research nurse, two paediatric consultants, a paediatric respiratory/intensive care consultant, a public health consultant, a general practitioner, a health economist, and a patient representative.

Inevitably, there will be professional groups involved in patient care who cannot be represented on the guideline development group. In the example above there is no physiotherapist, no radiologist and no otolaryngologist. The reason why not everyone can be on the GDG is simple: committees with more than about 12 participants become unmanageable. A line has to be drawn somewhere.

This does not mean, however, that professional groups not included on the GDG should have no say in the guideline. It just means they have to be included in other ways (see 'Stakeholder involvement' below).

Selection

How do you choose an individual to be on the GDG? The gold standard method is practised at NICE.[7] They have established collaborative groups from different backgrounds and specialties. When a new guideline is started, they ask these groups to nominate a member to be on the GDG. In this way, the GDG is independently selected and is not simply made up of friends of the guideline co-ordinator.

In most cases, however, these resources are not available. So basically you have to approach potential volunteers.

Tips

Identifying GDG members

Regional guidelines	Invite members from all parts of the region to be on the GDG.
	If the GDG is made up of only Trust 'A' employees, no-one in Trust 'B' will be motivated to use the final guideline.
National guidelines	Look through the websites of national professional bodies (e.g. Royal College of Nursing) and find the person responsible for clinical effectiveness/guidelines. Ask them to be on your GDG or, if they can't, get *them* to nominate someone else.
	For bodies without a named person for clinical effectiveness, write to the chief executive officer and ask them to nominate someone.

Don't be surprised if your potential field of volunteers is small. You will need to explain what the commitment involves (how many meetings, over what timescale and what level of background input is expected) and what the benefits will be to them.

Recruiting and retaining GDG members

Demonstration of continuing professional development (CPD) is required by many colleges for revalidation of their members.

• Being a member of a GDG counts towards CPD.

Travel to meetings can be an obstacle for potential GDG members.

• Use email groups to discuss issues if individuals can't attend meetings.
• Use conference telephone calls (if resources allow).

A GDG ideally needs to be balanced with experts and front-line staff.

■ A guideline written purely by eminent professors may not be in tune with what front-line staff can deliver or what patients expect.

■ A guideline written purely by practitioners with only a superficial knowledge of a topic may result in the 'partially sighted leading the blind'.

Note: a GDG does not organize itself spontaneously. Whoever is co-ordinating the guideline will inevitably have to organize the agendas and timetables for meetings.

Patients

The views of patients are both important and valid. In guideline development, it is easy to forget that it is the patient whom we are really developing the guideline for. The patient representative on the GDG will focus the guideline on the patient not the providers, the treatment or the cost.

Example Box 4.4

NICE, when developing the NICE guideline on Caesarian section,[8] included two 'consumers' (patient representatives) on their GDG. Recommendations were made from evidence relating to prognosis, and therefore risk in various circumstances. When making judgements about risks to mothers and babies, the views of mothers need to be included. Without their views discussed, the GDG would have been guessing at what patients wanted – the paternalistic approach of old.

The final recommendations included all the various perspectives, including those of the consumers.

NICE have a Patient Involvement Unit and Citizens' Council to provide patient representation for their guidelines. To recruit patients try the Royal Colleges, who have lay representatives. Also, ask members of charities/patient support networks related to the guideline's topic or the Patient Advice and Liaison Service to contribute.

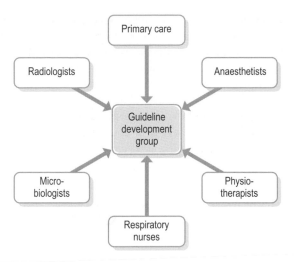

Figure 4.1 Some of the stakeholder groups contributing to the 'Breathing difficulties' guideline[6] developed by the Paediatric Accident and Emergency Research Group.

Stakeholder groups

As mentioned previously, not all professional bodies can be represented on the GDG. To ensure that these potential end-providers of the guideline's recommendations have input in the development process, there must be open channels of communication, so their opinions can be heard and influence the final guideline (Figure 4.1).

Identifying members of stakeholder groups can be even harder than identifying members for the GDG. Ask the GDG members to form links with affiliated specialties (e.g. use the respiratory physician on the GDG to liaise with respiratory nurses and physiotherapists) or to help identify key people to contact. Again, websites of national professional bodies can be a useful source of information. Patients are also stakeholders, so again recruit from the Royal Colleges, charities/patient support networks or the Patient Advice and Liaison Service.

> **Tips**
>
> **Recruiting stakeholder groups**
> Identify one member of a national body as a link to the GDG. Ask that link to liaise with their colleagues in the whole organization – the stakeholder group.
> Document the names of these links, their stakeholder group and their contributions.

What do the stakeholders have to do?

They should be asked to comment on each stage of the guideline development, from its initial scope to its final format. The stakeholders often bring up questions related to the scope of the guideline, which hadn't been thought of initially. They can highlight research which had not been found in the evidence searches (see Chapter 6: Searching for evidence). They can help answer specific questions, which only those practising in that field can answer. They can contribute to the consensus process for the guideline (see Chapter 8: Consensus processes). Finally, they can externally appraise the guideline before and/or after final publication.

The process of gathering a representative GDG and identifying potential stakeholder groups can take 2–3 months by the time all the links have been identified and they have agreed to participate. Why go to all this trouble? The reason is twofold and again is related to the idea of 'beginning at the end':

1. *Appraisal.* The final guideline will be assessed on its level of stakeholder involvement.

2. *Free advertising.* The more people who know about and are involved in the guideline, the easier it will be to disseminate the final product when written.

Scoping the guideline

The scope of a guideline is probably the most important, and most difficult, aspect of guideline development. It must clearly define to whom the guideline is meant to be applied (i.e. the guideline is aimed at which patients and at what point in the disease process/journey through the health system), to whom the guideline is not meant to be applied (i.e. special cases or grey areas where the recommendations won't apply), in which areas will recommendations be made by the guideline (i.e. what are the clinical questions which will be answered by the recommendations) and at what point does the guideline finish (i.e. at what point in the patient journey is the last clinical question to be answered by the recommendations).

To whom does the guideline apply?

You've already started to think about this when bringing together the GDG. Carefully define the patient population to whom you want the final guideline to apply.

1. Define the illness/condition/problem for which the guideline is being developed.

2. Define inclusion and exclusion criteria for the following patient characteristics:
   - age of patients;
   - new patients/chronic patients;
   - severity of illness;
   - special cases or conditions surrounding the problem;
   - other conditions which the patient may have.

3. Define the healthcare setting where the guideline is to be used and the health professionals expected to use the guideline

The issues above can usually be identified readily and agreement reached by the guideline development group at the first meeting.

Example Box 4.5 NICE hypertension guideline[9]

Definition of hypertension
- Persistently raised blood pressure above 140/90 mmHg

Patient characteristics included/excluded from the guidance
- For adults
- Guidance for newly identified patients with hypertension
- Severe hypertension (BP >160/100 mmHg) included in guideline
- Excludes secondary hypertension (high blood pressure related to renal, pulmonary, endocrine or other underlying disease)
- Includes patients with existing coronary heart disease or diabetes

Healthcare setting
- General practice
- Management in the hospital setting is not covered by guideline

---

In which areas will recommendations be made?

This part of the scope of the guideline can be very hard to define and may take longer. Basically, which treatments will be reviewed by the guideline and which treatments will be left outside the remit of the guideline.

Look carefully at your patient's journey. Along the way, what treatment options may be offered by various professional groups? Is there a pecking order to the treatments (i.e. first line, second line, etc.)? Is there a timescale within which certain treatments are offered?

Example Box 4.6

NICE 'Self-harm' guideline[10]	The guideline makes recommendations which cover the first 48 hours following an act of self-harm, but does not address the longer term psychiatric care of people who self-harm.
NICE Hypertension guideline[9]	The guideline makes recommendations which cover diagnosis, lifestyle changes for patients with hypertension and drug therapies including thiazide diuretics, betablockers, calcium-channel blockers, ACE inhibitors and angiotensin-receptor blockers in primary care. Further treatments were outside the scope of the guideline.
SIGN 66 Childhood otitis media in primary care guideline[5]	The guideline makes recommendations which cover diagnosis, antibiotics, decongestants, antihistamines, mucolytics, analgesics, oils, steroids, auto-inflation and homoeopathy. Further treatments, including surgery, were outside the scope of the guideline.

Make a list of the available treatments and discuss them one by one with the GDG. Drawing a draft algorithm for the guideline, before the evidence search has started or any recommendations have been made, may help the GDG define the start, middle and end of the guideline (Figure 4.2).

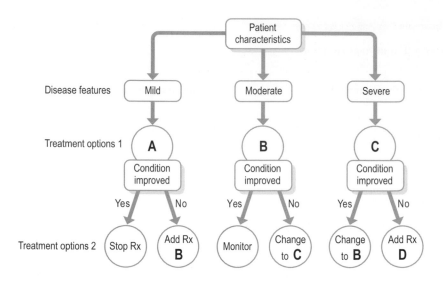

Figure 4.2 Example of a draft algorithm to help define the scope of the guideline.

If the scope is too wide, the project will never be finished. If the scope is too restrictive, then target-users may feel that the guideline doesn't address the questions they really want to know the answers to.

If a treatment is not offered in the healthcare setting where the guideline is to be used (e.g. a surgical procedure in a primary healthcare setting), then it is probably outside the scope of the guideline. If a treatment is available in some but not every healthcare setting where the guideline is to be used, then that treatment probably should be looked at (to determine whether it should be recommended as a valuable treatment across the NHS or not). The recommendations in the guideline need to follow the patient's journey. Therefore, if first-line therapies and third-line therapies are to be included in the guideline, then second-line therapies also have to be included, otherwise there will be a hole in the final guideline.

Refining the scope

Once the GDG has discussed the draft scope of the guideline initially, ask for comments from the stakeholder groups. They will come up with further special cases/ conditions that need to be included or excluded from the guideline, and they will suggest different aspects of the scope which hadn't originally been discussed.

During the evidence searching and literature reviewing, further aspects of the topic will come to light and these will need to be addressed to be either included in or excluded from the final guideline.

The final scope should fulfil the objectives of the guideline and cover the relevant questions in that particular field. Getting the scope completely right from the outset is unlikely to happen. If the scope evolves during the development process then ensure that the reasons for it changing are clearly documented.

Summary

- Read the AGREE Instrument.
- Document the reasons for selecting the guideline topic.
- Assemble a guideline development group with links to other stakeholders.
- Discuss the scope of the guideline and refine it if necessary.

References

1. The AGREE Collaboration. Appraisal of guidelines for research and evaluation (AGREE Instrument). 2001. www.agreecollaboration.org.
2. NICE: About clinical guidelines. National Institute for Clinical Excellence, London, 2004. www.nice.org.uk.
3. SIGN 50: Selection of guideline topics. Scottish Intercollegiate Guidelines Network, 2004. www.sign.ac.uk.
4. Armon K, Stephenson T, Gabriel V et al. Determining the common medical presenting problems to an accident and emergency department. Arch Dis Child 2001; 84:390.
5. SIGN: Diagnosis and management of childhood otitis media in primary care. Guideline No. 66. Scottish Intercollegiate Guidelines Network, 2003. www.sign.ac.uk.
6. Lakhanpaul M, Armon K, Eccleston P et al. An evidence based guideline for the management of children presenting with acute breathing difficulty. 2003. Nottingham: Paediatric Accident and Emergency Research Group. www.nottingham.ac.uk/paediatric guideline/breathingguideline.pdf
7. NICE: Guideline development methods – Chapter 4: Forming and running a guideline development group. National Institute for Clinical Excellence, London, 2004. www.nice.org.uk.
8. National Institute for Clinical Excellence. Caesarian section. NICE Clinical Guideline No. 13. 2004. London: National Institute for Clinical Excellence. www.nice.org.uk
9. National Institute for Clinical Excellence. Hypertension: Management of hypertension in adults in primary care. NICE Clinical Guideline No. 18. London: National Institute for Clinical Excellence. 2004. www.nice.org.uk.
10. National Institute for Clinical Excellence. Self-harm: The short-term physical and psychological management and secondary prevention of self-harm in primary and secondary care. London: National Institute for Clinical Excellence. 2004. www.nice.org.uk.

Chapter 5

Forming clinical questions

Richard Bowker

Aims

- To identify the importance of clinical question selection and formation
- To describe how to ask a question in an answerable form
- To provide useful tips to avoid pitfalls in question formation

Stimulation for developing a guideline often comes from clinical events where the recurrent question 'What should I do in this situation?' has an ill-defined answer. Guidelines try to answer these clinical questions in a way that will influence practice for the better. Therefore, the ability to ask the right questions will determine in part the success of the guideline.

Anyone can ask a question. However, many questions about clinical practice are poorly formed and therefore rarely generate a satisfactory answer. Guideline developers should spend time at the beginning of the process generating the precise questions they are trying to answer for the guideline user.

Selecting and constructing clinical questions

Thoughtful question formation will help with:

- scoping the guideline;
- focusing the evidence searches;
- determining important outcomes when forming recommendations.

Scoping the guideline

This has already been mentioned in the previous chapter but getting the scope right cannot be stressed enough if the guideline is to be a manageable project. After the guideline topic has been chosen, the guideline development group (GDG) should consider what is known in this area to help define the guideline's boundaries.

Once the population, disease parameters, beginning and end-points of the guideline have been decided upon (see 'Scoping the guideline' section in Chapter 4), the GDG should ask:

- What are the key clinical questions which need answers?
- What clinical questions are diversions from the main topic of the guideline?

The questions will be very different if they are drawn up by doctors compared to patients, or by nursing staff compared to health economists. Thus, a long list of questions may initially be drawn up and discussed, but the GDG must be sure that the ones which are finally selected make the guideline useful and usable at the end.

Look at the clinical questions posed by the NICE guideline developers on 'Depression'[1] (see below). The guideline was aimed at general practitioners as well as hospital psychiatrists. If a GP was confronted by a patient with depression, would most of the important questions the doctor or patient asks be covered by this guideline? Are there any major questions which are omitted? Or are any questions irrelevant?

Example Box 5.1 Clinical questions answered by the NICE guideline on depression

Pharmacology questions:
1. Is any single (or class of) antidepressant better than others in the treatment of depression?
2. Does the choice of antidepressant depend on: severity of depression?
    depression sub-type side effects?
    discontinuation symptoms?
    setting?
    gender?
    age?
3. What pharmacological strategies are effective in refractory depression?
4. Is St John's wort effective in depression: by severity of depression?
    compared to antidepressants?
5. Which switching strategies are effective?
6. What are the best pharmacological management strategies to prevent relapse?

Psychology questions:
1. Are psychological interventions effective compared to: treatment as usual?
    other psychological interventions?
    medications?
2. Is there a benefit in combining psychological interventions with medication?

Service questions:
1. Does screening for depression by GPs improve outcomes?
2. In depression, does guided self-help improve outcomes compared to other interventions?
3. Does computerized cognitive behavioural therapy improve patient outcomes compared to other treatments?
4. Does exercise improve patient outcomes compared to other treatments?
5. In depression, which model of care produces the best outcomes?
6. Do non-statutory support groups improve outcomes?
7. Do crisis resolution and home treatment teams improve patient outcomes compared to other treatments?
8. Do day hospitals improve patient outcomes compared to other treatments?
9. Does electroconvulsive therapy improve patient outcomes compared to other treatments?

Using the example above, most of the GP's questions would be answered regarding treatment, whether pharmacological or non-pharmacological. Some questions would be irrelevant for the GP, but they might be very pertinent to the hospital psychiatrist for intervention or service development.

The scope of the guideline has been defined by the questions which the guideline tries to answer.

Focusing the evidence searches

Defining the questions clearly at the beginning:

- reduces the number of searches you have to perform;
- helps with the search strategies;
- assists with the selection of articles for review.

The overall number of evidence searches needed to be performed will be determined by the number of clinical questions the GDG has selected. If irrelevant questions are included, then valuable time will be used on fruitless searches.

Once the questions selected have been dissected into answerable forms (see 'How to form an answerable question' below), it will become easier to identify the ideal type of study required to find the answer. They will also provide several of the key words to input into the literature databases, e.g. Medline, Embase, Cochrane (see Chapter 6).

When looking through the abstract titles generated by a literature search, referring back to the original question will help to keep you – the literature reviewer – focused on the selection of potentially relevant articles (see Chapter 6). It is all too easy to be captivated by an interesting yet totally unrelated abstract and waste time during a search with distractions.

Relating recommendation formation to important outcomes

When forming the answerable clinical question (see 'How to form an answerable question' below), part of the question will relate to the outcome which the GDG feel is clinically relevant.

Example Box 5.2 NICE guideline: depression

Clinical question:
Is any single antidepressant better in the treatment of depression?

Before the search for the evidence can begin, the GDG will have to decide what is meant by 'better' in terms of a clinically relevant outcome.

Does a clinically relevant outcome for the treatment of depression mean:
- a significant difference in suicide rates over 6 months?
- a significant reduction on a depression score at 6 weeks?
- no difference between resolution of depression but a difference in side-effect profile?

If the evidence which is found reported the selected clinically relevant outcome and demonstrated a beneficial effect, then recommendation for the use of that treatment or service can clearly be made. If the evidence available used a different outcome measure, then this surrogate marker may or may not be clinically relevant. This will impact on the strength of the recommendation which can be made about that treatment.

By the GDG agreeing on relevant clinical outcomes early in the guideline development process, recommendation forming is not only easier but also transparent (see Chapter 11).

How to form an answerable question ('framing questions')

Questions come in many forms. They can be roughly divided into background questions and foreground questions.

■ Background questions ask for general knowledge about a condition. They usually are made up of two components: a question root (e.g. what, where, who, when, why, how) and a disorder. An example of a background question would be, 'What is pneumonia?'. The answers to background questions are often found in general textbooks rather than research papers.

■ Foreground questions ask for more specific information about diagnosis, prognosis, therapy, harm or causation. They are usually made up of three or four components:

- • a population of patients
- • an intervention
- • a comparison
- • an outcome

this is a 'PICO' question

An example of a foreground question about therapy would be, 'In children with pneumonia diagnosed by an X-ray [population], does treating with intravenous penicillin [intervention] compared to oral amoxicillin [comparison] reduce the time to recovery measured by hospital stay [outcome]?'. Finding the answers to foreground questions when developing guidelines will require a literature search and review.

Foreground questions initially start life as vague statements (see examples below). From these vague questions, a more specific question needs to be formed to target the answer we are looking for. The way in which a question is formed is determined by the type of information being sought, whether that be related to diagnosis, prognosis, therapy, harm or causation.

Example Box 5.3 Vague foreground questions for a guideline on meningitis in children

What is the best test for children with suspected meningitis?
What is the prognosis for children with a diagnosis of meningitis?
What is the best treatment for children with meningitis?
Are there any risks associated with vaccinating against meningitis?

Once a question is structured, the next steps are literature searching (Chapter 6), evidence appraisal (Chapter 7) and finally recommendation formation (Chapter 11) to answer the original question.

Questions of diagnosis

In real life, confidence in a diagnosis is a continuum from uncertainty to absolute certainty. Our opinions change as more information becomes available. After taking a history we may still be uncertain about the exact diagnosis but a potential list is drawn up. This list is hopefully reduced by examining the patient. Finally, investigations are performed to improve the certainty of one diagnosis over another.

Note: history or clinical findings are considered to be 'investigations', as they can be positive or negative in exactly the same way a blood test/X-ray can be.

The questions generated around diagnosis try to ascertain how much certainty is gained by performing a test, asking a question, finding a clinical sign or a combination of these methods. To determine this we have to know what conditions need to be met to make the diagnosis as certain as possible. This is usually the 'gold standard' diagnostic test. All other tests need to be compared with this 'gold standard' to see how they match up, i.e. how much certainty will they provide compared to the current best diagnostic certainty.

A diagnostic question can be formed from three parts:

■ a population with a suspected condition;

■ the candidate test being positive (or negative) in that population (often labelled 'exposure' by convention in evidence-based medicine circles);

■ the outcome of having the condition or not by comparing with 'gold standard' testing.

(This does not fit into the 'PICO' format, but for standardization 'PECO' has been coined.)

Each part of the question needs to be specific to what is really being asked. Several specific questions may be generated from one vague question, but the chances of answering the specific questions will be much higher.

43

Example Box 5.4

Initial question:
• What is the best test for children with suspected meningitis?

Population	By 'children' do you mean any person from preterm infants to 18-year-olds?
	Do you want to divide the population into different age groups, e.g. 0–1 year, 1–5 years, etc.?
	By 'suspected meningitis', do you mean 'meningitis' written in the notes by the responsible practitioner or did you want to define this by specific physical signs being present, e.g. neck stiffness, temperature, headache, etc.?
	What type of meningitis are you interested in: bacterial; viral; tuberculous?
Investigation or 'Exposure'	Which investigation are you interested in: a clinical sign?
	a blood test?
	cerebrospinal fluid (CSF) microscopy?
	How is a positive test defined: a clinical scale?
	a threshold on a distribution curve?

Continued

Example Box 5.4 *Continued*

Outcome	What is the 'gold standard' diagnostic test for meningitis?
	Assessment of each case by a panel of experts
	Positive polymerase chain reaction result from CSF
	Positive culture result from CSF

Final framed questions:
- In children aged 5–12 years with a stiff neck, temperature and headache [population], and with a C-reactive protein level of less than 100 mg/L [exposure], what is the chance that they have bacterial meningitis diagnosed by a positive CSF culture or positive CSF polymerase chain reaction result [outcome]?
- In children aged 5–12 years with a stiff neck, temperature and headache [population], and with a CSF microscopy with less than 20×10^9 white blood cells per mm^3 [exposure], what is the chance that they have bacterial meningitis diagnosed by a positive CSF culture or positive CSF polymerase chain reaction result [outcome]?

By using the final framed questions in the example above, the guideline will answer the relevant clinical questions:

- If a practitioner suspects meningitis, do they need to perform a relatively invasive lumbar puncture if, on a blood test, the C-reactive protein is less than 100 mg/L?

- If a practitioner suspects meningitis but the initial CSF microscopy has fewer than 20×10^9 white blood cells per mm^3 do they need to start antibiotics or can they wait for the culture result 24 hours later?

Evidence

The types of papers which will help to answer these questions are studies using a blind comparison of the candidate test with the validated 'gold standard' test. Remember that a 'test' can be a history finding, a clinical finding or a laboratory/radiological finding.

The recommendation will be based on whether the test in question generates enough certainty about the diagnosis to be relied upon or not.

Questions of prognosis

Patients will ask about their future health and health professionals have to understand the natural history of disease processes to advise them on treatment options. A structured prognosis question is made up from three parts:

- population;
- exposure to a condition;
- outcome.

Each part again needs to be specific, so the question can be answered with satisfaction by a literature review.

Example Box 5.5

Initial question:
• What is the prognosis for children with a diagnosis of meningitis?

Population   Do you want to divide the population into different age groups, e.g. preterm
           infants on a neonatal unit, 0–1 year, 1–5 years, etc.?
           Do you want to include children with venticulo-peritoneal shunts?

Exposure   By meningitis do you mean bacterial, viral or tuberculous meningitis?
           Did you want to specify an organism, e.g. meningococcus or pneumococcus?
           Is late presentation/treatment relevant to the outcome?
           Is the part of the world where they present important?

Outcome   Are you interested in mortality in the first few days or weeks?
           Are there any complications of the disease which do not manifest themselves
           until much later but which are clinically relevant?

Final framed questions:
• In children aged 0–12 months [population], with a confirmed diagnosis of pneumococcal meningitis in the United Kingdom treated within 24 hours of symptom onset [exposure], what is the
risk of death or bilateral deafness after 1 year [outcome]?
• In children aged 0–12 months [population], with a confirmed diagnosis of pneumococcal meningitis in the UK presenting a week after first symptoms [exposure], what is the risk of death or
bilateral deafness after 1 year [outcome]?

Evidence

Questions of prognosis are best answered with prospective population-based cohort studies.

Prognostic information in a guideline may be useful for communication with patients per se. It can also denote risk factors or subgroups within the population, which should be treated more aggressively or referred for specialist care early.

However, prognostic questions will not always help with recommendation forma-tion. Therefore, the GDG should think carefully about how searching for this infor-mation will help the end-user of the guideline.

Questions of therapy

Patients should be offered the best treatment available for their condition. Structured questions of therapy are made up with four parts:

- population;
- intervention;
- comparison;
- outcome.

Example Box 5.6

Initial question:
• What is the best treatment for children with meningitis?

Population   By 'children' do you mean any person from preterm infants to 18-year-olds?
           What type of meningitis are you interested in: bacterial; viral; tuberculous?

Continued

Example Box 5.6 *Continued*

Intervention	Which treatment are you interested in: a specific antibiotic?
	the addition of steroids?
	Is there a specific length of treatment which needs to be defined?
Comparison	Ideally, a placebo would be the comparison treatment but there would be ethical difficulties with this approach for meningitis.
	What is the standard treatment currently used for the condition?
Outcome	Is the mortality rate the only outcome which will satisfy your question?
	Which elements of morbidity are clinically important to patients?

Final framed questions:
- In children aged 5–12 years with a diagnosis of pneumococcal meningitis on CSF culture or PCR [population], does treating with dexamethasone 0.4 mg/kg twice a day for 2 days in addition to normal antibiotic therapy [intervention] compared to placebo in addition to normal antibiotic therapy [comparison] reduce the incidence of bilateral hearing loss [outcome]?
- In children aged 1–12 years with a confirmed diagnosis of pneumococcal meningitis [population], does treatment with once-daily intravenous ceftiaxone for 7 days [intervention] compared to four times a day benzylpenicillin for 14 days [comparison] result in an increased incidence of bilateral hearing loss [outcome]?

By using the final framed questions in the example above, the guideline will answer the relevant clinical questions:

■ if a practitioner suspects pneumococcal meningitis, should they add dexamethasone therapy to the antibiotic regime?

■ if a practitioner confirms pneumococcal meningitis, will a shorter course of antibiotics be detrimental to the clinical outcome, assuming that there are desirable non-clinical benefits of a reduced stay in hospital?

Evidence

The ideal types of papers to help answer these questions will be randomized controlled trials (RCTs) or, even better, systematic reviews of RCTs.

The recommendations for therapy will be based primarily on whether a beneficial effect is shown with the candidate treatment. However, an analysis of harm of the therapy and any cost implications should also be taken into account (see Chapter 10: Health economics).

A similar approach to question formation can be used for questions about preventative therapies.

Questions of harm and causation

Exposure to a therapeutic agent or an environmental factor may cause harm. An estimate of the likelihood of this harmful event occurring is required to weigh up the balance of benefits and risks associated with treatment.

Structured questions of therapy are made up with four parts:

■ population;

■ exposure;

Example Box 5.7

Initial question:

- Are there any risks associated with vaccinating children against meningitis?

Population	By 'children' do you mean any person from preterm infants to 18-year-olds? What type of meningitis are you interested in: bacterial; viral; tuberculous?
Exposure	Which specific vaccination are you interested in: HiB? MenC? Mumps? Pneumovax?
Comparison	The group not exposed to the vaccine should be similar to those given the vaccine.
Outcome	Is the mortality rate the only outcome which will satisfy your question? Which elements of morbidity are clinically important to patients? What is the appropriate time period of follow-up for the outcome to be detected?

Final framed question:

- In children vaccinated before 6 months old [population], does administering the conjugated pneumococcal vaccine [intervention] compared to placebo [comparison] lead to an increased incidence of developmental delay diagnosed by the age of school entry [outcome]?

- comparison (not exposed);
- outcome.

Using the example above, the final framed question will help answer:

- Is there a risk of developmental delay associated with vaccinating against pneumococcal infections per se (note: developmental delay is a recognized outcome in patients with pneumococcal meningitis)?

Evidence

An RCT has been heralded as the best evidence for establishing associations between exposure and harm, because confounding factors have been controlled for. However, even RCTs involving thousands of patients will not pick up rare adverse reactions and the follow-up length may be too short for detecting delayed effects. There may be ethical considerations preventing participants from being randomly exposed to potential harm. Cohort studies are the next best type of study, but again may not have the numbers to detect rare events. Finally, case–control studies are very good for looking at rare events, but conclusions about causation need to be carefully scrutinized for confounding factors, which cannot be controlled in this type of trial. Other evidence from phase IV studies (post-marketing surveillance), voluntary reporting schemes (e.g. the 'yellow card' system) or targeted reporting schemes (e.g. the British Paediatric Surveillance Unit reports) may be readily available. However, incorporating these data into a recommendation can prove difficult, as it is not considered to be 'strong' evidence (see Chapter 11: Making recommendations).

When appraising evidence of harm, it can be difficult to determine how the exposure and harm are related. Is the finding mere coincidence? Is there an association? Or is there evidence of causation? Often more than one source of evidence will be required to demonstrate causation,[2] including evidence of biological plausibility.

The evidence alone will not provide the answer for therapy questions where the balance between benefits and harms is evenly weighted. This is where patient preferences and values come into play. The GDG when forming therapeutic recommendations should be transparent about where the evidence came from for both risks and benefits, and how value judgements have been incorporated (see Chapter 11).

Tips for question forming

- Write down the current practice for the condition, which is the topic of the guideline. It is best to think of the patient journey from presentation to diagnosis, from initial treatment to second-line treatments.
- Every time there is a test or a treatment in this algorithm, which you have just written, there is an opportunity to ask a question. Is this the best test/treatment for this patient at this time in their management? Decide what the alternatives might be, and there you have the beginnings of a question to be answered.
- Ask the GDG and stakeholders to comment on these draft questions, and you will receive a number of unexpected but very useful responses.
- You will need to cull the number of questions before you start the evidence search. Be brutal! Many of the questions will be interesting but won't lead to useful clinical recommendations. Think about what the end-user of the guideline wants to know.
- Document the questions which have been selected. If during the course of guideline development further questions need to be answered, or previously selected questions become superfluous to the guideline, then document the reasons why the changes have been made and ensure that the GDG is in agreement.
- Questions of prognosis rarely lead directly to recommendations. Recommendations tend to be focused around therapy and diagnostic questions.

- Select the questions to form the scope of the guideline.
- Discuss the questions with the stakeholder groups.
- Frame the questions into an answerable form for diagnosis, prognosis, therapy, or harm.
- Refer back to the questions when forming the recommendations.

References

1. National Institute for Clinical Excellence. Depression. Management of depression in primary and secondary care. London: National Institute for Clinical Excellence. 2004. www.nice.org.uk
2. Raina P, Turcotte K. Assessing harm and causation. In: Moyer V, ed. Evidence based pediatrics and child health. London: BMJ Books; 2000, p 46–55.

Chapter 6

Searching for evidence

Richard Bowker

Aims

- To describe the process of translating a clinical question into a search strategy
- To suggest useful search strategies
- To explain the value of having inclusion and exclusion criteria before searching
- To point out the limitations in the process

49

At last you can get online and look for the evidence which is out there. Be warned – searching can be a tedious and laborious task. Preparation will save you time and frustration.

Before you start:

- List the clinical questions the guideline development group (GDG) has agreed upon for the guideline (see Chapter 5: Forming clinical questions).

- Group them into questions relating to therapy, diagnosis, prognosis and harm. Searches for therapeutic studies are generally easier than for prognostic information, so prioritize your searches by performing the easiest first.

- Write out a timetable for the searches. This way you should know which searches have been completed and how many more are to be done.

- Prepare a filing system for searches and papers.

- Ask for help from the library staff – they may even do the searches for you!

- Decide how exhaustive the systematic search needs to be to satisfy the guideline's questions.

Translating a clinical question into a search strategy

Look carefully at the clinical question. Break it down into its component sections of population, intervention/exposure, comparison, and outcome (see Example Box 6.1).

Example Box 6.1 Guideline: Management of depression in primary and secondary care[1]
Type of question: Therapy

Question	[Population] In adults with newly diagnosed depression,
	[Intervention] do SSRI antidepressants
	[Comparison] compared to tricyclic antidepressants
	[Outcome] improve depression scores significantly more at 6 weeks?
Keywords	Depression, antidepressants, selective serotonin re-uptake inhibitors, tricyclic
Trials	Systematic review of RCTs, RCTs

In each part, you should be able to find a key word or words. These will be used to form part of the search strategy.

Next, think about what type of question you are answering: therapy, diagnosis, prognosis or harm. This will aid the development of a search filter.[2]

Search strategies

When the guideline is published, reviewers will want to be confident that a systematic search for evidence has taken place. They will want to know where and how the search took place, and the method by which the papers were chosen or discarded. There are no set rules here. Look at the AGREE Instrument (Appendix 1) to determine whether you feel you will be appraised favourably on the methods you plan to use. Make it clear in the final guideline document what actions were undertaken during the searches, so that the process can be repeated by someone else.

Where to search

Electronic

There is a long list of specialized databases of medical research (Table 6.1). Which databases to search should be based on the topic of the guideline and where the relevant literature is likely to be indexed.

Cochrane is freely available through the NLH (National Library for Health – www. library.nhs.uk), as is MEDLINE (although you may prefer to access this through Ovid rather than through Entrez PubMed). Many other search engines can also be accessed through NLH but require you to hold an Athens account. This facility is free for all NHS employees, so speak to your hospital library if you don't have one. Many other databases can be accessed through university libraries.

The more search engines you use, the more likely you will be to find all the available evidence. The minimum to search would be Cochrane, MEDLINE and EMBASE (this covers the majority of the world's medical/biological publications).

How far back do you need to search?

This is never an easy question. Some of the most established practices are based on poor evidence from a long time ago. In these cases it is likely that you will have to go

Table 6.1

Specialized databases	
Cochrane Library	A register of systematic reviews and RCTs
MEDLINE	A register of all types of published trials run by the US National Library for Medicine (1966 onwards)
EMBASE	A register of all types of published trials run by a European based publishing house
British Nursing Index	A register of all types of published trials focusing on nursing specialties
CINAHL (Cumulative Index to Nursing and Allied Health Literature)	A register based in the USA (1983 onwards)
PsycINFO	A register run by the Americal Psychological Association (1974 onwards)
AMED (Allied and Complementary Medicine Database)	A register of complementary medicine papers
The list goes on …	

back as far as the databases allow. Evidence on the latest treatment, however, is much more likely to have been published recently. So you could limit the search to the last 12 years or so.

Hand search

It is useful to look through the references of the papers you select for appraisal to see if there are other papers that may be relevant. It may also be revealing to hand search the last 12 months of the most respected journals in the field, as electronic searches can miss key papers.

Stakeholders

Ask if they are aware of any data that may answer the clinical questions being asked.

Unpublished trials

Publication bias means that journal editors are more likely to publish positive results, with negative or equivocal results not reaching the public domain. Unpublished data may be held by drug companies, the UK Medicines and Healthcare Products Regulatory Agency (MHRA), the US Food and Drug Administration (FDA) or European Medicines Agency (EMEA). These agencies may claim that the data are confidential but invoking the UK freedom of information act may precipitate a response.

Searching for unpublished trial data is very time consuming and rarely rewarding. If you have resources to do this, concentrate on finding data for therapy questions.

Remember: 'systematic' does not mean 'exhaustive'. A search could go on for ever if you want to read every journal ever published! Provided the search strategy is logical, well documented and thorough, the appraisal should be positive.

How to search

It is very difficult to explain how to use the various online databases in a book, and therefore we shan't try!

Key knowledge – not delivered by this book – to acquire for searching includes:

■ how to use medical subject heading (MeSH) terms;

■ how to combine search terms;

■ how to save your searches permanently.

If you have difficulty with finding your way around MEDLINE, Cochrane or EMBASE, ask your local library for a tutorial. They will usually be most obliging. PubMed also has a range of online tutorials, which are easy to run through.

The rest of this chapter assumes that you have some knowledge of using electronic databases.

Search filters

Electronic literature searching is not an exact science! Ideally, you would like a search strategy to identify all the papers which are totally relevant (a sensitive search), and to disregard all the papers which are unrelated to the question of interest (a specific search). We are looking for a perfect 'search filter'. No such thing exists!

Filtering using keywords of the question

The purpose of a systematic search in guideline development is not to miss any evidence, so the search needs to be wide rather than targeted (sensitive rather than specific). It is therefore useful to use medical subject heading (MeSH) terms in combination with text word terms.

MeSH terms may find the same number of papers as the text words typed into the database. They often find more papers or sometimes they find fewer papers. In Example Box 6.2 you will not be criticized by narrowing the search to those papers only related to type 1 diabetes, as the question is specific for this population. However, the MeSH term 'blood glucose' has found nearly 20 times more papers than 'glycaemic control'. Combining the two terms using the OR option, there are now 24 535 hits. This proves that the two terms do not totally overlap. It is therefore worthwhile playing with different text words and MeSH terms to get the right combinations.

Example Box 6.2 Building a search strategy using MeSH headings

Question	In adults with newly diagnosed type 1 diabetes, what type of initial insulin regime gives best glycaemic control?		
Keywords	**Hits using text words alone**	**MEDLINE MeSH terms**	**Hits using MeSH terms**
'Adult'	870 158	'Adult'	870 158
'Diabetes'	84 190	'Diabetes mellitus, type 1'	15 854
'Insulin'	31 492	'Insulin'	31 492
'Glycaemic control'	1 304	'Blood glucose'	23 828

Unfortunately, different databases may use slightly different subject headings. So each search needs to be done individually for each database (or include multiple subject headings, combining them with OR).

If there is no such MeSH term available, then searching for text words within the paper or abstract is required.

Remember to think of different spellings of the same word and combine them with OR (e.g. paediatric OR pediatric).

Also, different endings of words can be overcome by using a wildcard symbol (e.g. 'hyperglycemi$' searches for the terms 'hyperglycemia' and 'hyperglycemic'). This wildcard symbol is a dollar sign $ if using Ovid MEDLINE or an asterisk * if using PubMed MEDLINE.

Filtering using the type of question being asked

Simply using the keywords from the clinical question will probably generate thousands of titles to look through. Adding a filter (Table 6.2) for the type of clinical question being asked may reduce this number somewhat. Simply type in the search filter – exactly as written in the right-hand column of Table 6.2 – into PubMed MEDLINE and combine it with the key text words or MeSH terms, and that will be your search strategy. (For an explanation of the parentheses, colons and asterisks look in the 'Help' section of PubMed under 'PubMed Character Conversions' – although this level of understanding is not really required.)

The filters in Table 6.2 have been tested only in MEDLINE and are not transferable, as the syntax will be different in other databases (i.e. EMBASE does not recognize all the terms used in MEDLINE). Filters for use in other databases are less well

53

Table 6.1

Filters for optimizing searches for different types of clinical questions[3–6]

Question type	Sensitivity of search filter	Specificity of search filter	Search filter for PubMed MEDLINE
Therapy	99%	70%	((clinical[Title/Abstract] AND trial[Title/Abstract]) OR clinical trials[MeSH Terms] OR clinical trial[Publication Type] OR random*[Title/Abstract] OR random allocation[MeSH Terms] OR therapeutic use[MeSH Subheading])
Diagnosis	98%	74%	(sensitiv*[Title/Abstract] OR sensitivity and specificity[MeSH Terms] OR diagnos*[Title/Abstract] OR diagnosis[MeSH:noexp] OR diagnostic*[MeSH:noexp] OR diagnosis,differential [MeSH:noexp] OR diagnosis[Subheading:noexp])
Harm	93%	63%	(risk*[Title/Abstract] OR risk*[MeSH:noexp] OR risk *[MeSH:noexp] OR cohort studies[MeSH Terms] OR group*[Text Word])
Prognosis	90%	80%	(incidence[MeSH:noexp] OR mortality[MeSH Terms] OR follow up studies[MeSH:noexp] OR prognos*[Text Word] OR predict*[Text Word] OR course*[Text Word])

validated and not easy to find. You will have to create your own with text words or MeSH terms similar to those in Table 6.2. Another source of filters can be found on the SIGN website (www.sign.ac.uk/methodology/filters.html).

Even with these search filters in place, there will be a large number of irrelevant papers which will slip through the net. This is merely a result of how the papers have been indexed. The lot of a guideline developer is not an easy one!

Combining search terms

Combining the terms is quite simple.

- OR e.g. 'meningitis' OR 'encephalitis'; the results of this search will include papers which mention either meningitis or encephalitis, or both.

- AND e.g. 'meningitis' AND 'encephalitis'; the results of this search will include only those papers which refer to both meningitis and encephalitis. If only one is mentioned it won't be included.

- NOT e.g. 'meningitis' NOT 'encephalitis'; the results of this search will only include papers which refer to meningitis alone. If encephalitis is also mentioned in the paper, this paper will not be included.

Combining terms can dramatically reduce the number of papers in a search. Don't be tempted to combine too many terms together using AND. If you end up with no papers to search through, undo the last combination and consider searching each term independently.

Limiting the choice of papers

Inclusion and exclusion criteria

Look again at the original question. What type of paper are you looking for? Which population are you interested in? Which interventions are key to the question? When looking through the papers always keep your mind on what question you are trying to answer.

Titles

You may end up with 100 to 10 000 titles to look through. If you have 10 000, consider refining your search filters again, as you will be amazed at what has slipped through!

Focus your mind on the original question again and skim-read all the titles. Choose the ones which match the selection criteria (type of study, population, type of intervention). Any titles which may be related to this question should also be selected for further examination. Do not select any papers which relate to other questions in the guideline during this search. Do not select papers which catch your eye but are totally off the topic – your personal learning agenda will only slow down the process!

Abstracts

From the selected titles review the abstracts. Filter out any papers which do not fit the selection criteria when examined closely. Be ruthless! There are a lot of grey data out there which will not contribute to the levels of evidence or grades of recommendations found.

What about the papers which don't have abstracts published?

■ This is a difficult question. How do you know whether an interesting title is really the key piece of evidence you've been looking for, or just another case report pretending to be an RCT! Some searchers would select these papers and read through them. Others may be pragmatic and say that due to limited resources these titles were not chased up. Decide and document how you will deal with these titles.

What about foreign-language papers?

■ Publication bias comes into play here. All journal editors prefer to publish positive results. Good studies, which show equivocal results, will often be rejected by the major journals, which are almost always published in English, but may be picked up by the less well known journals publishing in other languages. Therefore, papers in foreign language journals may demonstrate different results to those available in English. However, most guideline developers don't have the translating services of the United Nations available to them. Each paper costs about £100 to translate. Many guideline developers take the view that foreign-language papers should be searched for (i.e. titles selected and abstract reviewed), but due to limited resources they cannot be translated and therefore do not become part of the evidence base. By documenting the titles of the foreign-language papers you would have liked to review but were unable to, the whole selection process remains transparent.

Articles to read

Having selected a number of articles from the abstracts, go and locate them. This may take longer than the expected trip to the local library as you may need to wait for interlibrary loans to be processed. Photocopy the article twice so that you have one copy to read and one to file safely. The article can still be rejected at this stage if it doesn't reach the entry criteria or it can be excluded on other grounds. However, now that it has been read you must document why you rejected it at this stage.

Appraisal of individual papers and evidence tables will be dealt with in Chapter 7.

Pitfalls in searching

Searching the wrong questions

You are unlikely to find evidence in the literature to help make specific recommendations about clinical definitions, routine observations or routine investigations. Ask yourself at the beginning of the process, which searches will be fruitful and which will be fruitless. Decide with the GDG which recommendations will not be based

Example Box 6.3 A documented search strategy[7]
Specific treatments for children with herpes simplex encephalitis

Background
Children who have a reduced conscious level may have herpes simplex encephalitis (HSE). The treatment of HSE with antiviral medication may improve outcome in children. Is there evidence that treatment of suspected cases of HSE improves mortality and neurological morbidity in children?

Question
For children with HSE, does treatment with aciclovir compared to any other treatment improve the mortality and neurological morbidity?

Paper selection criteria
Inclusion criteria were drawn up before the search took place. Papers were selected if they were randomized controlled trials of antiviral treatments for HSE, with concealment of randomization, and if outcome measures included mortality and neurological morbidity. Papers which studied adults and children would be included, as the treatment effects would be likely to cross the age range. Papers in foreign-language journals would be included in the search and referenced but not included in the final selection of papers due to limited translation facilities.

Search strategy
A review of the Cochrane Library, MEDLINE (1966–present), EMBASE (1980–present), CINAHL (1982–present), British Nusing Index (1985–present) and AMED (1985–present) was performed in April 2004. The search terms can be reviewed below. A review of the references of the selected papers for further evidence was included in the search strategy. Authors of included papers were contacted to clarify any uncertainties in the research methodology.

#	Search history	Results
1	RANDOMIZED CONTROLLED TRIAL.pt.	188702
2	CONTROLLED CLINICAL TRIAL.pt.	66249
3	randomized controlled trials.sh.	33319
4	random allocation.sh.	50966
5	double blind method.sh.	78357
6	single blind method.sh.	8068
7	or/1-6	320919
8	clinical trial.pt.	392544
9	exp clinical trials/	493355
10	(clin$ adj25 trial$).ti,ab.	201983
11	((singl$ or doubl$ or trebl$ or tripl$) adj25 (blind$ or mask$)).ti,ab.	154873
12	placebos.sh.	25805
13	placebo$.ti,ab.	170336
14	random$.ti,ab.	565198
15	research design.sh.	39333
16	or/8-16	1277257
17	comparative study.sh.	1171853
18	exp evaluation studies/	517733
19	follow up studies.sh.	283694
20	prospective studies.sh.	204144
21	(control$ or prospectiv$ or volunteer$).ti,ab.	2743177
22	or/17-21	4266411
23	7 or 16 or 22	4861234
24	exp infant, newborn/ or exp infant/ or exp infants/	923566
25	exp adolescent/ or exp adolescence/ or exp adolescent, hospitalized/	1388009

Continued

Example Box 6.3 *Continued*

#	Search history	Results
26	exp child/ or exp children/ or exp child, preschool/ or exp childhood/ or exp child, hospitalized/	1 585 340
27	24 or 25 or 26	2 739 385
28	23 and 27	711 510
29	aciclovir.mp. [mp=ab, hw, ti, sh, it, tn, ot, dm, mf, rw]	15 525
30	acyclovir.mp. [mp=ab, hw, ti, sh, it, tn, ot, dm, mf, rw]	11 455
31	29 or 30	22 407
32	28 and 31	1 039
33	encephalitis.mp. [mp=ab, hw, ti, sh, it, tn, ot, dm, mf, rw]	31 656
34	exp encephalitis/	44 202
35	33 or 34	53 293
36	32 and 35	105
37	vidarabine.mp. [mp=ab, hw, ti, sh, it, tn, ot, dm, mf, rw]	5 740
38	28 and 37	219
39	36 and 37	39

Search results

From 144 titles, a total of 17 abstracts were reviewed.
From a hand search of the references a further 5 abstracts were reviewed.

Three papers were selected for review from the abstracts.[1-3]

Skoldenberg et al (1984) and Whitley et al (1977) were included. Whitley et al (1986) was excluded as concealment of randomization could not be guaranteed.

1. Whitley R et al. Adenine arabinoside therapy of biopsy-proved herpes simplex encephalitis. N Engl J Med 1977; 297(6):289–294.
2. Skoldonberg B et al. Acyclovir versus vidarabine in herpes simplex encephalitis. Randomised multicentre study in consecutive Swedish patients. Lancet 1984; 2(8405):707–711.
3. Whitley R et al. Vidarabine versus acyclovir therapy in herpes simplex encephalitis. N Engl J Med 1986; 314(3):144–149.

on published evidence, but will be based on expert opinion (see Chapter 8). This will save a number of searches and therefore valuable time.

Search filters

There is no 'correct' search filter to use. None is perfect. The number of case reports which you trawl through, despite actively trying to filter them out, is infuriating. It is probably not worth spending too much time trying to design the perfect filter. Use a simple filter and resign yourself to searching through reams of titles.

Computers

One of the most time-saving but also frustrating aspects of searching is using a computer. Being in the middle of a long search only for the web server to crash is very disheartening.

Always back up the work which has been done. Don't leave the entire guideline on one computer or in one file. Two years of work can easily be lost if the hard drive fails! Keep updated versions on CD-ROMs, different servers, different computers, etc.

Database updates

Hypothetical scenario. You have completed your search through the titles and you have selected the abstracts. You decide to save this search before looking at the abstracts in detail and have a 15-minute break. The abstracts are saved as a list of numbers, which correlate to the order of the titles you've just spent an hour looking through. While you are away the database updates, and a few new papers are added. All the titles in the search are shifted, which means all the abstracts you selected bear no relation to the ones you wanted! You have to start from scratch again.

Moral of this 'hypothetical' scenario:

- complete a whole search in one go;
- print out the results (titles and abstracts of chosen papers, and their references);
- save the search and write it up, before going for your break!

Not finding any useful evidence

Unfortunately this is often inevitable. Current practice is often based on experience rather than good published evidence. If you don't find any evidence out there, don't blame yourself. It probably isn't there! Don't repeat the search five times over. Document the search (see Example box 6.3) and move on to the next one.

Summary

- Choose the databases for searching (minimum of Cochrane, MEDLINE, EMBASE).
- Use the clinical question to develop the search strategy.
- Ask for help from librarians to develop search filters.
- Use the clinical question to focus the selection process.
- Be ruthless with the exclusion criteria (grey data are not helpful on the whole).

References

1. National Institute for Clinical Excellence. Depression: Management of depression in primary and secondary care. NICE Clinical Guideline No. 23. London: National Institute for Clinical Excellence. 2004. www.nice.org.uk
2. Hunt D et al. Finding the evidence. In: Moyer V et al, eds. Evidence based pediatrics and child health. London: BMJ Books; 2000.
3. Haynes R et al. Developing optimal search strategies for detecting clinically sound studies in MEDLINE. J Am Med Inform Assoc 1994; 1(6):447–458.
4. Wilczynski N et al. Developing optimal search stragtegies for detecting clinically sound prognostic studies in MEDLINE: an analytic survey. BMC Med 2004; 2(1):23.
5. Haynes R et al. Optimal search strategies for retrieving scientifically strong studies of diagnosis from Medline: analytical survey. BMJ 2004; 328(7447):1040.
6. Montori V et al. Optimal search strategies for retrieving systematic reviews from Medline: analytical survey. BMJ 2005; 330(7482):68.
7. The Paediatric Accident and Emergency Research Group. The management of a child with a decreased conscious level. 2005. www.nottingham.ac.uk/paediatric-guideline

Chapter 7

Critical appraisal and building evidence tables

Richard Bowker

- To describe the different systems available for levels of evidence
- To define the type of study in the paper being appraised
- To describe the appraisal tools available for individual study types
- To build an evidence table and assign levels to evidence

59

Introduction

You have spent several days searching for and retrieving papers to answer one of the clinically relevant questions developed by the GDG. Now you have to appraise the evidence which has been found.

You therefore have to be able to:

- appraise individual papers for their strengths and weaknesses;
- summarize each paper in an evidence table to help the group make recommendations;
- designate a level of evidence for each paper so that the end-users have an easy understanding of where this study sits in the hierarchy among other studies.

As with other parts of guideline development, you have to work backwards and first choose a system of evidence hierarchy before you start appraising individual papers (Figure 7.1).

Levels of evidence

Evidence can come from many different types of research. The guideline developer needs to be able to recognize and then convey to the end-user:

- What is strong evidence?
- What is average evidence?
- What is weak evidence?

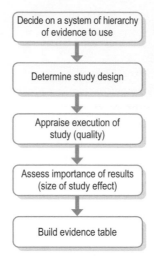

Figure 7.1 Summary of evidence appraisal for guideline developers.

In the past the answers to these questions were *assumed* to be simple:

- Strong evidence is published in high-quality peer-reviewed medical journals by a name everyone knows.

- Average evidence will be published in journals which no-one really reads, including non-English-language journals.
- Weak evidence remains unpublished.

This is *not* the case.

Journals publish papers primarily to sell journals. Publication bias is well documented.[1] Positive findings are far more likely to be published than negative or equivocal findings. Publication bias potentially overestimates any treatment effects or test accuracies.

Well known researchers have to continue to publish to remain 'well known' and secure funding. There are rare but high-profile cases of 'misrepresenting' the data in order to be published.[2]

Over the last 20 years those practising evidence-based medicine have developed and evolved hierarchical lists of evidence to determine which type of evidence is more likely to provide an answer closer to the truth than another. Unfortunately, there are now at least five different 'levels of evidence' systems in common use[3] (Table 7.1). All the systems have one thing in common: level or hierarchy of evidence is based on

1. the study design;
2. the study execution.

Hierarchy due to study design

Many guideline developers use a single classification system for all the clinical questions in the guideline. The classification system used by SIGN and NICE is shown in Table 7.2 and that used by the Agency for Healthcare Research and Quality (AHRQ) for the US National Guideline Clearinghouse in Table 7.3.

Commonly used classification systems for hierarchy of evidence

Classification system	Reference/source
Scottish Intercollegiate Guidelines Network	www.sign.ac.uk
American College of Chest Physicians	www.biomedcentral.com
Oxford Centre for Evidence-based Medicine	www.cebm.net
Australian National Health and Medical Research Council	www.nhmrc.gov.au/publications/synopses/cp65syn.htm
US Task Force on Community Preventive Services	www.thecommunityguide.org

Table 7.2

Levels of evidence based on type of study design used by SIGN and NICE[4]

Levels of evidence

1++	High-quality meta-analyses, systematic reviews of RCTs, or RCTs with a very low risk of bias
1+	Well conducted meta-analyses, systematic reviews of RCTs, or RCTs with a low risk of bias
1−	Meta-analyses, systematic reviews of RCTs, or RCTs with a high risk of bias
2++	High-quality systematic reviews of case–control or cohort studies
	High-quality case–control or cohort studies with a very low risk of confounding, bias, or chance and a high probability that the relationship is causal
2+	Well conducted case–control or cohort studies with a low risk of confounding, bias, or chance and a moderate probability that the relationship is causal
2−	Case–control or cohort studies with a high risk of confounding, bias, or chance and a significant risk that the relationship is not causal
3	Non-analytical studies, e.g. case reports, case series
4	Expert opinion

61

Table 7.3

Levels of evidence based on type of study design used by AHRQ[5]

Levels of evidence

I	Evidence from randomized controlled trial(s)
II-1	Evidence from controlled trial(s) without randomization
II-2	Evidence from cohort or case–control analytical studies, preferably from more than one centre or research group
II-3	Evidence from comparisons between times or places with or without the intervention; dramatic results in uncontrolled experiments could be included here
III	Opinions of respected authorities, based on clinical experience; descriptive studies or reports of expert committees

The classification systems in Tables 7.2 and 7.3 make life simple for both the appraiser and end-user – one type of study design always trumps another type, with the randomized controlled trial being the ace in the pack.

Unfortunately life is not quite that simple. The belief that the double-blind randomized controlled trial is the king of evidence no matter what the clinical question

Table 7.4

Levels of evidence based on type of clinical question (adapted from Phillips et al[6] with explanatory notes available from www.cebm.net)

Level	Therapy/prevention/aetiology/harm	Prognosis	Diagnosis	Differential diagnosis/symptom prevalence study	Economic and decision analyses
1a	Systematic reviews of RCTs	Systematic review of inception cohort studies; clinical decision rule validated in different populations	Systematic review of Level 1 diagnostic studies; clinical decision rule with 1b studies from different clinical centres	Systematic review of prospective cohort studies	Systematic review of Level 1 economic studies
1b	Individual RCT (with narrow confidence interval)	Individual inception cohort study with ≥80% follow-up; clinical decision rule validated in a single population	Validating cohort study with good reference standards; or clinical decision rule tested within one clinical centre	Prospective cohort study with good follow-up	Analysis based on clinically sensible costs or alternatives; systematic review(s) of the evidence; and including multi-way sensitivity analyses
1c	All or none before and after trials	All or none case series	Diagnostic test studies with 100% sensitivity or 100% specificity (Absolute 'SpPins' and 'SnSnouts')	All or none case series	Absolute better-value or worse-value analyses
2a	Systemic review of cohort studies	Systematic review of either retrospective cohort studies or untreated control groups in RCTs	Systematic review of Level <2 diagnostic studies	Systematic review of 2b and better studies	Systematic review of Level >2 economic studies

Table 7.4

Continued

2b	Individual cohort study (including low-quality RCT; e.g. <80% follow-up)	Retrospective cohort study or follow-up of untreated control patients in an RCT; derivation of clinical decision rule or validated on split-sample only	Exploratory cohort study with good reference standards; clinical decision rule after derivation, or validated only on split-sample or databases	Retrospective cohort study, or prospective cohort study with poor follow-up	Analysis based on clinically sensible costs or alternatives; limited review(s) of the evidence, or single studies; and including multi-way sensitivity analyses
2c	'Outcomes' research; ecological studies	'Outcomes' research		Ecological studies	Audit or outcomes research
3a	Systematic review of case–control studies		Systematic review of 3b and better studies	Systematic review of 3b and better studies	Systematic review of 3b and better studies
3b	Individual case–control study		Non-consecutive study, or without consistently applied reference standards	Non-consecutive cohort study, or very limited population	Analysis based on limited alternatives or costs, poor-quality estimates of data, but including sensitivity analyses incorporating clinically sensible variations
4	Case series (and poor-quality cohort and case–control studies)	Case series (and poor-quality prognostic cohort studies)	Case-control study, poor or non-independent reference standard	Case series or superseded reference standards	Analysis with no sensitivity analysis
5	Expert opinion without explicit critical appraisal, or based on physiology, bench research or 'first principles'	Expert opinion without explicit critical appraisal, or based on physiology, bench research or 'first principles'	Expert opinion without explicit critical appraisal, or based on physiology, bench research or 'first principles'	Expert opinion without explicit critical appraisal, or based on physiology, bench research or 'first principles'	Expert opinion without explicit critical appraisal, or based on economic theory or 'first principles'

is not true. For questions of intervention (i.e. Is one treatment superior to another treatment?) then an RCT is the best study (or better still a systematic review of lots of RCTs) to answer this query. However, for other types of clinical question an RCT may not be applicable. RCTs are poor at flagging up rare but serious side effects, for example. The 'best' type of study design for a particular question may be a cohort study (e.g. questions of prognosis). For this reason other classification systems[6] have been developed which base hierarchy on the type of clinical question being asked (Table 7.4).

Clearly, such a classification system is more complex to use. However, it does provide a more logical hierarchy for non-intervention questions. The level of evidence for a diagnostic test is often higher using the classification system in Table 7.4 than using the one in Table 7.2. Thus the end-user may have more confidence in using that test and therefore make implementation easier.

The decision to choose one classification system over another is in the end quite arbitrary (see Table 7.1 for options). If the guideline you are developing is concerned mainly with therapeutic interventions, then a simple system will be more than adequate. Whichever system is chosen, it should be used throughout the guideline and described clearly in the methodology to keep the process transparent.

Determining the study design

Bearing in mind that part of the appraisal of evidence is based on the study design, it is reasonable to spend a bit of time looking into how you can tell what type of study you are appraising. It may seem obvious, as many studies will state this in the abstract. However, what is stated and what actually happened can often be two different things.

The algorithm in Figure 7.2 will help you to determine what type of study you are appraising and Example Box 7.1 explains what each type of study is.

Interpretation is especially difficult for the observational studies.

- When does a case series differ from a retrospective cohort study?

- What type of study assesses the accuracy of diagnostic/screening tests?

- What about studies which look at the agreement between groups of professionals assessing clinical features?

Case series and cohort studies

Many studies reported to be cohort studies are indeed case series. The difference between a retrospective cohort study and a case series is subtle.

A case series is a collection of patients who have all had the same procedure or disease.

- Recruiting patients is performed retrospectively by looking through databases.

- The timescale for recruiting participants into a case series is usually many years.

- The population from which the cases are selected is often quite narrow, e.g. one unit's caseload, and not all the cases may be identified. In this way the results will not be widely applicable to other populations.

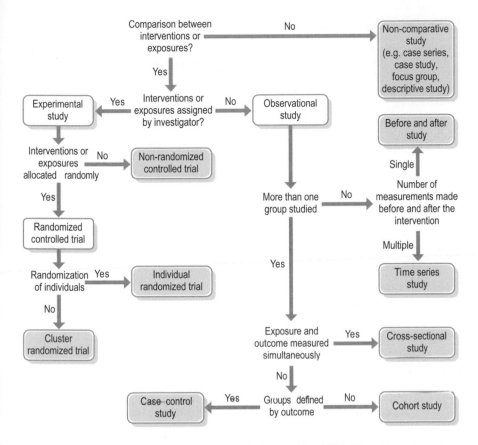

Figure 7.2 Algorithm to determine the type of study design (adapted from NICE – The guidelines manual 2006[7]).

65

- Case series will often report on the differences between patients who had a good outcome and a poor outcome, making the study look similar to a cohort study.
- A case series gives no information about the rates of disease in the general population.

A retrospective cohort study is reported in the same way as a prospective cohort study (comparing rates of outcomes between exposed and unexposed populations) but the recruitment into the cohort is performed after the outcome *not* before.

- The population may be identified from an existing cohort used for a prospective study or by using an established population database.
  - For example, a study looking into the rates of breast cancer in women who breast-fed their offspring compared to those who didn't breast-feed collected data on this population for 15 years. A new study wanted to look at the rate of bowel cancer in women who ate meat compared to vegetarians. They used the same cohort, as the information was available on rates of bowel cancer and diet in the population.

Example Box 7.1 Description of study types

Experimental studies
Some study conditions are under the control of the investigator to reduce confounding factors.

Study design	Definition
Randomized controlled trial	Participants randomly assigned to intervention or control group, with a comparison of outcome rates over the study period. Randomization avoids selection bias because both known and unknown confounding factors are on average equally distributed between the two groups.
Non-randomized controlled trial (quasi-experimental study)	Allocation of participants to different intervention groups is controlled by the investigator but not in a truly random manner.

Observational studies
The investigator reports findings without any control over the study condition.

Study design	Definition
Cohort study	Outcomes of participants who have been exposed to a condition or intervention are compared with a group who were not exposed in a follow-up study. The allocation of participants is not controlled by the investigator.
Case-controlled study	Rates of exposure to a condition or intervention in a group with a known outcome (cases) are compared with the rates of exposure in a group who did not have the outcome (controls).
Cross-sectional study	Study of the relationship between disease and other factors as they exist in a population at a single point in time.
Before and after study	Study comparing participants before and after an exposure or intervention.
Case series	Description of a number of participants undergoing an intervention or having a condition with no comparison of a control group.

- The population is ideally recruited over a limited timescale.
- As the population is not the same as the general population then the applicability of the results will be reduced but not to the same extent as in a case series.
- The study will report rates of outcomes in the two cohorts (exposed/unexposed).
- Retrospective cohort studies can provide evidence of rates of disease in populations.

Diagnostic tests

In the simple systems of evidence hierarchy, a comparison of a new diagnostic test compared with a gold standard test would be classed along with cross-sectional studies or cohort studies. The more sophisticated classification systems provide more information on how the study can be appraised (see Table 7.4.)

Agreement between groups

The fact that a diagnostic test exists does not mean it is useful. Often a test requires a large degree of subjective interpretation. If this interpretation differs greatly between individuals then the accuracy of the test will be highly operator-dependent (e.g. performing part of a clinical examination or performing an ultrasound scan). There are several studies which look at the agreement of individuals when performing the same test on the same patient.

Neither the simple nor the more sophisticated hierarchy systems can place these studies. Generally they are classed along with cohort studies although there is no official consensus on this matter. Perhaps this highlights the fact that very few recommendations are based solely on these types of studies.

Determining the study quality

The design of the study you are appraising has now been classed as a meta-analysis, an RCT, a cohort study, a case–control study, a diagnostic test study or a case study. Next you have to appraise how well the study was executed. Whole books have been devoted to the appraisal of different studies[8,9] and therefore to try to summarize this in a chapter is impossible.

Several reports have looked at which factors in study design produce the most accurate results and which factors are likely to produce erroneous results by the introduction of bias.[10] From these reports, a variety of appraisal checklists have been developed which can be used to aid the appraisal process. If the guideline development group are using more than one appraiser of the selected papers, then it is useful for both to use a checklist. This way, disagreements in interpretation can be resolved quickly.

Questions of intervention

Randomized controlled trials quality assurance checklist

1. Was randomization to intervention groups adequate?
   - Adequate: computer-generated random numbers
                 random number tables
   - Inadequate: alternate numbers, dates of birth, days of week
2. Was allocation concealment adequate?
   - Adequate: centralized or pharmacy-controlled randomization
                 serially numbered identical containers
   - Inadequate: alternate numbers, dates of birth, days of week
                 open random number lists
                 serially numbered envelopes (even if sealed)
3. Were groups similar for disease prognosis at baseline?

4. Were inclusion and exclusion criteria specified?

5. Was the patient blinded to treatment allocation?

6. Were the healthcare professionals blinded to the treatment being provided?

7. Was treatment allocation blinded from the outcome assessors?

8. Were patients treated similarly apart from the intervention in question?

9. Was the follow-up of patients long enough and complete?

10. Were the primary outcome results reported?

11. Did the analysis include intention to treat?

Systematic reviews quality assurance checklist

1. Is this a systematic review of randomized controlled trials?

2. Is there an adequate methods section?
   - Adequate: description of finding the studies
     pre-determined inclusion criteria
     assessment of validity of individual studies
   - Inadequate: limited search for studies
     inclusion criteria not well defined
     studies not well scrutinized

3. Were the results consistent from study to study and was any heterogeneity explained?

Questions of prognosis, harm or causation

Cohort studies quality assurance checklist

1. Has a representative sample of patients been recruited at a common point in the disease process?

2. Is the 'exposure' reliably identified in the cohort?

3. Are the groups comparable on all important confounding factors and adjustments made?

4. Was follow-up long enough for the outcome to be measured?

5. What proportion of the cohort was lost to follow-up?
   - Adequate: <5%
   - Inadequate: >20%

6. Was outcome assessment objective and blind to exposure status?

Case–control studies quality assurance checklist

1. Is the case definition explicit?

2. Have the cases been reliably assessed and validated for disease state?

3. Have the controls been randomly selected from the source population of the cases?

4. Have controls been matched on factors which are unrelated to exposure?
5. Were exposures measured in the same way for both cases and controls (objective measure or assessment of exposure blinded from outcome)?
6. Did the exposure precede the outcome?
7. Is there a dose-related response?
8. Does the association make biological sense?

Questions of diagnosis

Diagnostic test studies quality assurance checklist
1. Was the diagnostic test evaluated in a population of patients in whom there was diagnostic uncertainty?
2. Was there an independent and blind comparison with a reference ('gold') standard for the diagnosis in question?
3. Was the 'gold' standard test performed in all patients regardless of the result of the candidate diagnostic test?

Further checklists can be found in SIGN 50[11] and the NICE guidelines manual 2006.[7]

Unfortunately, many studies published before the 1980s do not mention in the methodology the required appraisal criteria. It may be that their methods were flawed or that they didn't report exactly what they did, as it was not a pre-requisite to getting published. Contacting the lead authors to find out what they did would be the gold standard solution. However, resources and time are likely to be an issue and therefore this may not be possible in reality. Luckily in the post-CONSORT[12] era, methodology write-ups are generally more thorough, making appraisal of modern papers much easier.

Once the study design and quality have been assessed, the level of evidence can be assigned.

Size of study effect

If the study design or quality is poor then the size of the study effect is not that important, as it will be flawed. However, the size of study effect is the next important step in evidence appraisal when the design and quality are appraised as good.

Study results are reported using a number of different statistical definitions. When looking at a number of studies it is useful to standardize the reporting of results for the evidence table. Again, below is only a very brief introduction into the world of medical statistics. Further reading is strongly advised.

Intervention

An intervention study may report the treatment effect by:
- number needed to treat;
- relative risk;
- relative risk reduction.

It should be possible to convert results from all the studies into a number needed to treat (NNT = the number of patients needed to be treated to benefit one patient) by using the following formulas:

■ Absolute rate reduction (ARR) = Control event rate − Experimental event rate

■ $\text{NNT} = \dfrac{1}{\text{ARR}}$

(Control event rate = the number of adverse events in the control group; experimental event rate = the number of adverse events in the intervention group.)

■ Relative risk $= \dfrac{\text{Experimental event rate}}{\text{Control event rate}}$

An examination of the confidence intervals of the relative risk is important. If they cross 1 then there is no statistical difference in outcomes between the treatment and control group.

For example, if in an RCT of 200 obese men aged 50 to 55, there were 10 myocardial infarctions over a 5-year period in the control group (n = 100) but only 5 in the experimental group (n = 100) who underwent a 2-week 'obesity reduction programme' at the start of the trial, then:

■ $\text{ARR} = \dfrac{10}{100} - \dfrac{5}{100} = \dfrac{5}{100} = 0.05$

■ $\text{NNT} = \dfrac{1}{0.05} = 20$ patients would need to be treated to reduce the number of myocardial infarctions by 1

■ Relative risk $= \dfrac{\frac{5}{100}}{\frac{10}{100}} = 0.5$ (i.e. you are half as likely to have a myocardial infarction if you have the intervention)

However, look at the confidence intervals (not given in this example).

Prognosis

A prognostic study will report the risk of an event occurring over a set period of time.

There is no way of standardizing the results which report events occurring over different timespans.

Harm

Ideally all results are reported as the number of treatments/exposures needed to harm one patient (number needed to harm – NNH). However, it depends how the study has been designed. Harm data can come from RCTs, cohort studies or case–control studies. Case–control studies need to be analysed differently as the number of outcomes is controlled, not the size of the cohorts.

		Adverse outcome		Totals
		Present (case)	Absent (control)	
Exposed	Yes (cohort)	a	b	a + b
	No (cohort)	c	d	c + d
	Totals	a + c	b + d	a + b + c + d

In an RCT or cohort study:

Control event rate (CER) $= \dfrac{c}{c + d}$

Experimental event rate (EER) $= \dfrac{a}{a + b}$

$NNH = \dfrac{1}{CER - EER}$

In a case–control study: Odds ratio (OR) $= \dfrac{a \times d}{b \times c}$

$$CER = \dfrac{c}{c + d}$$

$NNH = \dfrac{CER \times (OR - 1) + 1}{CER \times (OR - 1) \times (1 - CER)}$

Diagnosis

A diagnostic test study may report the accuracy of the test by:

- sensitivity and specificity;
- positive and negative predictive values;
- likelihood ratios;
- risk ratios.

		Disease		Totals
		Present	Absent	
Test	+ve	a	b	a + b
	−ve	c	d	c + d
	Totals	a + c	b + d	a + b + c + d

Sensitivity $= \dfrac{a}{a + c}$

Specificity $= \dfrac{d}{b + d}$

$$\text{Positive predictive value (PPV)} = \frac{a}{a + b}$$

$$\text{Negative predictive value (NPV)} = \frac{d}{c + d}$$

$$\text{Likelihood ratio for a positive result} = \frac{\text{Sensitivity}}{1 - \text{Specificity}}$$

$$\text{Likelihood ratio for a negative result} = \frac{1 - \text{Sensitivity}}{\text{Specificity}}$$

$$\text{Risk ratio positive result} = \frac{\text{PPV}}{1 - \text{NPV}}$$

$$\text{Risk ratio negative result} = \frac{1 - \text{PPV}}{\text{NPV}}$$

Sensitivity and specificity are not affected by the prevalence of the disease in the study population, whereas PPV and NPV are. Therefore sensitivities and specificities or likelihood ratios can be used to compare study results.

For example, the gold standard test for a urinary tract infection is a positive urine culture from a mid-stream urine sample. This takes 24 hours to come back from the laboratory. A leucocyte dipstick test costs less and gives an immediate result. In a study, the leucocyte test was positive 220 times in 230 positive urine cultures, and was positive in 7 of 100 negative urine cultures.

Therefore:

test+ disease+ = 220

test− disease+ = 10

test+ disease− = 7

test− disease− = 93

$$Sensitivity = \frac{220}{(220 + 10)} = 96\%$$ (i.e. if disease is present then the test will be positive 96% of the time)

$$Specificity = \frac{93}{(7 + 93)} = 93\%$$ (i.e. if disease is absent then the test will be negative 93% of the time)

$$PPV = \frac{220}{(220 + 7)} = 97\%$$ (i.e. if test is positive then the disease will be present 97% of the time)

$$NPV = \frac{93}{(10 + 93)} = 90\%$$ (i.e. if test is negative then the disease will be absent 90% of the time)

Building evidence tables

Evidence tables are methodological, statistical and quality summaries of individual papers. They serve a number of purposes:

- summarize the evidence, so that the whole GDG does not need individually to appraise every single paper;

- allow direct comparisons of different papers to see how different conclusions may have arisen;

- aid in the production of a meta-analysis of the literature reviewed;

- provide the end-user with a means to look quickly at the evidence that helped develop the recommendations.

There are no strict rules on how to construct an evidence table and each type of study/clinical question will need a different format. Although NICE has a specific proforma for evidence tables for interventions and diagnosis, these are not widely adhered to as each GDG requests different information to be included. The example tables (Tables 7.5–7.8) are taken from a recent national guideline[13] to provide a flavour of what can be included.

Table 7.5

Example of evidence table for a therapy study/question[13]	
Study	Skoldenberg B, Alestig K, Burman L et al 1984 Acyclovir versus vidarabine in herpes simplex encephalitis. Randomised multicentre study in consecutive Swedish patients. Lancet 2(8405):707–711.
Methods	Randomized controlled muticentre trial in Sweden comparing vidarabine against aciclovir for the treatment of herpes simplex encephalitis (HSE).
Participants	Patients (aged over 4 weeks) with suspectd HSE and confirmed with brain biopsy for HSV immunofluoresence/ELISA/culture and/or CSF antibody levels against HSV. Study period March 1981 to July 1982.
Interventions	Aciclovir 10 mg/kg IV tds or vidarabine 15 mg/kg over 12 hours. Not blinded as difference in mode of delivery. All other treatments (inc. steroids) at the discretion of participating centre.
Allocation concealment	Randomization in blocks of 12 using sealed opaque envelopes.
Outcomes	Mortality and neurological sequelae at 6 months (no statement regarding primary/secondary outcomes or initial power calculation).
Results	127 patients with suspected HSE were enrolled and 53 of these had confirmed HSE. Of 53 patients, 27 were randomized to aciclovir. Of 27 aciclovir-treated patients 5 (19%) died compared to 12 of 24 (50%) vidarabine-treated patients – significant difference ($P = 0.04$). Two excluded from vidarabine-treated group as they relapsed and were started on aciclovir. 15/27 (56%) aciclovir-treated patients had no or minor sequelae at 6 months compared to 3/24 (13%) – significant difference ($P = 0.002$). No difference in moderate to severe sequelae between treatment groups.
Notes	During study period 5 cases of HSE were not enrolled – no reason given. Non-HSE group completed course of treatment with 2 deaths in 42 aciclovir-treated patients compared to 4/32 vidarabine-treated patients. No power calculation stated before study and no analysis in intention-to-treat groups for 2 dropouts in vidarabine group. The mortality rates in the vidarabine and aciclovir groups were similar to other studies. Drug toxicity was assessed during treatment with an erythematous rash noted in 1 aciclovir-treated patient and 12 moderate but transiently elevated alanine aminotransferase levels.
Evidence level	Therapy 1b.

Table 7.6

Example of evidence table for a systematic review[13]

Study	Prasad K, Singhal T, Jain N, Gupta P 2004 Third generation cephalosporins versus conventional antibiotics for treating acute bacterial meningitis (Cochrane Review). In: The Cochrane Library, Issue 3. Chichester, UK: John Wiley.
Methods	Systematic review of trials of intravenous antibiotics used for bacterial meningitis, comparing third-generation cephalosporins to other antibiotics.
Inclusion criteria	Eligible studies were published or non-published randomized controlled trials in which a third-generation cephalosporin was compared to the conventional treatment in patients with acute bacterial meningitis.
Search	Cochrane Central Register of Controlled Clinical Trials (CENTRAL), MEDLINE, and EMBASE were reviewed. Unpublished material also searched for.
Evidence appraisal	Two independent appraisers. They considered concealment of randomization, blinding, completeness of follow-up and intention-to-treat analysis.
Summarizing evidence	Meta-analysis provided including tests for homogeneity. Important outcomes included death and neurological sequelae.
Results	18 studies included (the majority of which were paediatric studies). No heterogeneity was found. There was no significant difference between using a third-generation cephalosporin and conventional antibiotics which covered a broad spectrum of bacterial pathogens.
Notes	Absence of evidence of an effect does not equal evidence of absence of an effect.
Evidence level	Therapy 1a.

Table 7.7

Example of evidence table for a prognosis study/question[13]

Study	Corey L, Rubin R, Hattwick M. 1977 Reye's syndrome: clinical progression and evaluation of therapy. Pediatrics 60(5):708–714.
Methods	Case series of patients with Reye's syndrome in USA.
Participant definition	Children (ages not defined) reported to the Centers for Disease Control in the USA with Reye's syndrome (meeting specific clinical criteria). The patients were then split according to different treatment groups and different illness severity. Study period December 1973 to June 1974.
Length of follow-up	To hospital discharge.
Outcomes	Death or neurological impairment at discharge.
Results	369 patients identified. 69% presented with stage 0–2/5 disease severity. A worse prognosis was seen in those patients whose blood ammonia level was greater than 300 mcg/dL (176 micromol/L) – mortality rate 27% vs 65% ($P < 0.001$).
Notes	This study demonstrates a relationship between plasma ammonia and outcome. However, collection of data was not uniform.
Evidence level	Prognosis 4.

Table 7.8

Example of evidence table for a diagnosis study/question[13]	
Study	Oostenbrink R, Moons K, Derksen-Lubsen G et al. 2004 A diagnostic decision rule for management of children with meningeal signs. European Journal of Epidemiology 19(2): 109–116.
Methods	Prospective validation study of a clinical diagnostic decision rule to determine the accuracy of a clinical test to detect bacterial meningitis in children.
Participants	Children (aged 1 month to 15 years) presenting to four centres in Holland with neck stiffness. Study period Nov 1999 to May 2001.
Diagnostic dilemma	Did the children with neck stiffness have bacterial meningitis?
Blinded comparison	The clinical decision rule was applied to them along with the gold standard of lumbar puncture (or follow-up to 1 week if no LP or antibiotics – i.e. no clinical deterioration in 1 week without treatment ruled out the diagnosis of bacterial meningitis).
Gold standard tested	Gold standard: CSF culture or no clinical deterioration without treatment within 1 week of presenting (if no lumbar puncture performed). Comparison test: clinical decision rule previously derived. (The rule included the following clinical features: duration of main complaint; vomiting; meningeal irritation; cyanosis; petechiae or ecchymoses; disturbed consciousness; serum CRP).
Results	Children with a score of less than 8.5 never had bacterial meningitis, while children with a score of more than 20 always had bacterial meningitis. Sensitivity of the test was 100% with a specificity of 60%.
Notes	The clinical signs and symptoms can be used for the diagnosis of bacterial meningitis. Bacterial meningitis is only one of several diagnoses which children who present with reduced conscious level have. During the study they reduced the cut-off value from 9.5 to 8.5 and did not re-validate prospectively. Therefore this is really a derivation study.
Evidence level	Diagnosis 2b.

Tip

After designing an evidence table for use in a guideline, get feedback from the GDG to make sure it contains enough information which is easily accessible and is fit for purpose.

Summary

- Select an evidence appraisal system to suit the guideline.
- Assess study design, quality and size of study effect in an objective manner.
- Summarize the evidence in evidence tables which meet the needs of the GDG and the end-user of the guideline.

References

1. Sutton A, Duval S, Tweedie R et al. Empirical assessment of effect of publication bias on meta-analyses. BMJ 2000; 320:1574–1577.

2. White C. Suspected research fraud: difficulties of getting at the truth. BMJ 2005; 331:281–288.
3. Atkins D, Eccles M, Flottorp S et al. Systems for grading the quality of evidence and the strength of recommendations I: Critical appraisal of existing approaches. The GRADE Working Group. BMC Health Serv Res 2004; 4:38.
4. Harbour R, Miller J. A new system for grading recommendations in evidence based guidelines. BMJ 2001; 323:334–336.
5. West S et al. AHRQ Publication No 02-E016. Rockville, MD: Agency for Healthcare Research and Quality; 2002. Systems to Rate the Strength of Scientific Evidence. Evidence Report/Technology Assessment No. 47; pp 64–88.
6. Phillips B et al. Levels of evidence and grades of recommendations. Oxford Centre for Evidence-Based Medicine. 1998. www.cebm.net/levels_of_evidence.asp
7. NICE. The guidelines manual 2006. www.nice.org.uk
8. Greenhalgh T. How to read a paper – the basics of evidence-based medicine. London: BMJ Publications, 2nd edn; 2002.
9. Sackett DL, Straus SE, Richardson WS et al. Evidence-based medicine: how to practice and teach EBM. 2nd edn. London: Churchill Livingstone; 2000.
10. Schulz KF, Chalmers I, Hayes RJ, Altman DG. Empirical evidence of bias. Dimensions of methodological quality associated with estimates of treatment effects in controlled trials. JAMA 1995; 273:408–412.
11. SIGN 50: A guideline developers' handbook. 2004. www.sign.ac.uk/guidelines/fulltext/50/index.html
12. Moher D, Schulz KF, Altman DG for the CONSORT Group. The CONSORT statement: revised recommendations for improving the quality of reports of parallel-group randomised trials. Lancet 2001; 357:1191–1194.
13. The Paediatric Accident and Emergency Research Group. The management of a child with a decreased conscious level. 2005. www.nottingham.ac.uk/paediatric-guideline

Chapter 8

Consensus processes
Kate Armon

- To determine when consensus is necessary
- To explain the different formal consensus methods available
- To discuss the validity of consensus in a guideline

Wouldn't it be great if all the clinical questions we asked were answered in the literature by large, valid, well conducted clinical trials yielding grade A recommendations? Wouldn't it also be great if the trial you found was conducted on the same population as yours (age, severity of illness, same disease definition/diagnostic test), used the same drug formulation/dose and was looking at the same clinically important outcome measures? Unfortunately we live in the real world where such research trials are rarely performed.

How do you generate recommendations for a guideline when there is a gap in the evidence base?

Consensus – when to use it in guideline development

If you are developing a guideline for use in a clinical setting that aims to direct clinicians on a pathway of care, you will find that there are areas where:

- there is no evidence[1-3] (see Example Box 8.1);

> **Example Box 8.1** Guideline 'Seizure – an evidence-based guideline for the management of children presenting post seizure'[4]
>
> The scope of the guideline was clearly defined, 18 clinical questions formulated, the literature search performed, papers found, critically appraised and recommendations graded (as in Chapters 4 to 7 of this book).
>
> However, of the 31 recommendations made, none was based on a grade A recommendation,[5] only 23% on a grade B (level 2++), 33% on C (level 2+) and 7% on D, leaving 37% with nothing in the literature at all on which to base the development of a recommendation.

- the evidence could lead to contradictory recommendations;
- the evidence does not completely relate to your patient group.

When faced with a gap in the evidence, a guideline development group (GDG) will be left with the following options:

1. Give no guidance. In the absence of evidence, any number of actions could be appropriate and clinicians should be left to their own knowledge, skills and judgements to decide what to do.
2. Audit current practices. The different ways patients are managed should be evaluated by audit so that the safest route can be determined.
3. Use an expert's opinion. In the absence of evidence, the 'best person' (expert) could be asked to advise on what to do.
4. Use the consensus of a group of practitioners. In the absence of evidence, a group of clinicians could be collected together to reach agreement on the way the patient should be managed in given circumstances.

Giving no guidance would mean that a junior practitioner, when seeing a patient with a condition with which he or she is unfamiliar, would either need to guess at what to do, surmise what to do after looking up the condition in a 'pocket book' (often expert opinion), or search on-line to find someone else's recommendations (very often inexpert opinion).

If an audit were performed to provide clues on the best course of action, it would be likely to take a long time to collect sufficient numbers. Even then the findings should be subjected to a randomized trial before they could be adopted as evidence based.

Using a single expert opinion is unlikely to inspire sufficient confidence in the guideline for its implementation to be successful! The problems with the 'expert' model are: first, defining who the best expert is; second, that this individual cannot be expected to be expert in all of the fields the guideline covers; third, that they may have limited credibility among the final guideline users.

The value of having several clinical experts contributing to and agreeing on a course of action should not be underestimated. They cannot provide 'grade A' recommendations (or even grade B or C!) but they will collectively arrive at a sensible, sound course of action. A group of individual 'experts' will have a wider range of experience and knowledge and should have more credibility when it comes to the acceptance of their collective judgement and its implementation.

Consensus can therefore be used to fill the gaps in the guideline left by a lack of clear evidence (Figure 8.1).

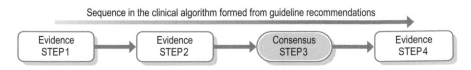

Figure 8.1 Using consensus as a stepping stone to create a coherent sequence of recommendations.

Consensus – when *not* to use it in guideline development

Having read this far into the book, you will be aware that guidelines must meet certain standards to be valid and result in any benefit to the patient. It is worth pointing out that this is a relatively recent development! Not so long ago many guidelines were produced by a panel of individuals (often 'experts') with poorly defined criteria for making decisions and giving pronouncements on clinical management.[6] During the 1990s the importance of validity and evidence in guideline development was emphasized.[1,7,8] Evidence-based guideline development now requires the explicit linkage of recommendations to the quality of the supporting evidence. This allows the user to make an informed choice about whether to comply with individual recommendations within the guideline depending on the quality of the supporting evidence.[6]

It is important to stress at this point, therefore, that consensus must never be used instead of strong evidence. The AGREE Instrument by which the guideline will be assessed is very clear that the recommendations should be evidence based. The Cochrane collaboration was formed because clear evidence from clinical trials was not making its way into practice in a timely way. Producing guidelines is one way of promoting the acceptance and adoption of good evidence. If consensus were to be used over and above evidence, the necessary changes in practice might never be achieved.

This can be a sticking point for a guideline development group. If the evidence clearly suggests that one form of practice is beneficial over another, then the better practice needs to be recommended, even if a consensus of practitioners prefer the other practice! Rigorous clinical research evidence trumps 'expert' opinion every time. This is not to say that clinical experience counts for nought, but that large-scale clinical trials are more objective than an individual's personal case series.

Consensus methodology

It is important to state clearly what a consensus process is and what it is not. It is a process for making policy decisions; it does not generate new scientific knowledge. Consensus development at best taps collective knowledge and at worst taps collective ignorance. However, even in the latter case, it can provide a marker of peer practice (see Chapter 15: Legal issues).

It will highlight areas of agreement and areas of disagreement. Where strong disagreement exists it can rarely resolve the dispute.[9] However, disagreement can be a useful tool for highlighting research priorities, where differences of practice exist based on limited evidence.

Informal consensus

The informal method involves gathering together a group of experts and allowing them to discuss the issue, with little information input and little structure to the discussion. The major problems with this approach are, first, that the group may become dominated by a vocal minority and, second, a tendency to try to enforce

79

unanimity, whereas the degree of dissent is in itself an important piece of information. Some cynics have called this method 'GOBSAT' (good old boys sitting around tables).

Formal consensus

To counter the problems of informal consensus more formal, systematic methods to harness 'expert' opinion have been developed. These have the advantage of being explicit, describable and repeatable, and thus tend to carry more authority and credibility. Such methods have been frequently used in the health field, although they themselves have been the subject of little methodological research (see 'Assessing the validity of consensus methods' later in the chapter). Many methodological issues therefore remain unresolved, and as a result there is no single, well defined established way to conduct consensus development.[10,11]

Nevertheless formal consensus is increasingly being used to develop guidelines.[12] If consensus is going to be used in the development of a guideline, informal methods should be avoided[13] as the formation of recommendations is not explicit.[2]

Methods of formal consensus development

- Nominal group technique
- Consensus conference
- Delphi technique

These three main approaches have been used in the health field. The RAND Corporation developed the Delphi method in the 1950s.[14,15] The nominal group technique followed this in the 1960s[16] and in 1977 the National Institute of Health in the USA introduced the consensus development conference.[17] Table 8.1 provides a schematic comparison of the three methods.

Table 8.1

Differences between consensus development methods			
	Delphi	**Nominal group technique**	**Consensus development conference**
Initial information given to participants	Yes (written)	Yes (written)	Yes (usually verbal presentation by experts)
Private decisions elicited	Yes	Yes	No
Formal feedback of group choices	Yes	Yes	No
Face to face contact	No	Yes	Yes
Interaction structured	Yes	Yes	No
Aggregation of results	Explicit (statistical)	Explicit	Implicit (qualitative, or simple majority vote)

The nominal group technique

The nominal group technique (NGT) has been widely applied in health and social services, education, industry and government organizations since its inception in the 1960s. The purpose of the NGT is to generate and rank ideas. The group is 'nominal' (in name only) in the sense that it is highly controlled and discussion is restricted to the later stages of the group process.[18]

First, each participant records his or her ideas independently and privately. The ideas are then listed in a round-robin format. One idea is collected from each individual in turn and listed by the group facilitator.[19] The participants then discuss each idea and individuals privately record their judgements or vote for options. Further discussion and voting may take place. Individual judgements are then aggregated statistically to derive a group judgement.

The developers argue that using this formal method, as opposed to an informal one, generates more ideas and discussion, rather than one or two ideas dominating. Because all participants are given space to contribute their ideas, the discussion is less likely to be dominated by one or two individuals. It requires a skilled facilitator.

A modified NGT commonly used for the development of clinical guidelines was developed by the RAND Corporation in 1992.[20] Initially individuals expressed their ideas privately through mailed questionnaires. The collated results of the questionnaire were fed back to each member of the group when they were brought together to discuss their views, after which they again privately recorded their views on a questionnaire.

It is thought that an NGT of 9–12 members is the maximum effective group size. Some researchers have run several groups in parallel, with feedback between groups as part of the process.

The consensus development conference

The US National Institutes of Health have run more than 100 consensus development conferences on a variety of topics.[21] The method has evolved with time and has been used in other countries including Canada, the UK (King's Fund) and Sweden.

A selected group of about 10 people is brought together for a meeting over several days. They hear evidence presented by various interested groups or experts. The meeting is chaired and questions can be asked throughout. The panel then retires to attempt to reach consensus, again with a chairperson managing the discussion. This type of conference is commonly beyond the means of most researchers (they cost approximately $90 000 each[21]) and is usually part of the defined programme of large organizations.

The Delphi method

This was developed by the RAND Corporation[14] to discuss the predictions for the effects of a nuclear war. Its name comes from the ancient Greek oracle at Delphi, who was believed to have the power to see the future. Its significant features are:

- anonymity;
- controlled feedback;
- iteration (the process occurs in rounds allowing individuals to change their view);
- and a statistical group response.[15]

In its original form (as used by the RAND Corporation), the first Delphi round consisted of a questionnaire based on a review of the evidence, which was sent to the panellists for comments. A modification of the first step is to include a preliminary round where individual panellists are invited to give their current opinion on a topic, based on their knowledge or experience. In the second and subsequent rounds (iteration), participants receive feedback on other group members' responses, and are given the opportunity to change their responses in the light of these. As it was first described, panellists were given statistical feedback only, but the method has been modified to include comments made by the participants. This is thought to elicit a more reasoned response.[22] The iterative rounds continue until either consensus is reached[19] (at a pre-defined level), stability occurs (no further change in panellists' responses between rounds), again at a pre-defined level, or the pre-determined number of rounds has been reached.

The vast majority of guideline development has been done with NGT or consensus development conferences. Delphi has tended to be used for prioritization of lists rather than for more complex issues. Nevertheless interest has increased in using Delphi for the development of clinical guidelines as its advantages are twofold. First, a larger number of people can be consulted, with no limit to the size of the group. In an NGT a maximum number of 9–12 panellists is recommended, but Delphi studies have been done with a range of participants (3 to 3000).[18] Guidelines produced with larger panels tend to be sound with high acceptability,[23] which will help with implementation later. Second, participants over a wide geographical area can be consulted without the expense of bringing them all together in one place. If you are aiming to produce a nationally acceptable guideline, geographic spread is important.

For all these reasons, the authors of this book have used the Delphi technique in developing guidelines. In the next chapter there is a detailed explanation on how to run a Delphi consensus process, based on what has worked well in the past.

Assessing the validity of consensus methods

Many methodological issues remain unresolved with formal consensus processes, which explains why there is no single, well defined, established way to conduct them.[10,11] However, there are ways in which it is possible to measure whether a consensus technique has come up with a valid 'answer', i.e. one which is closer to the best answer when compared to that given by an individual.

Murphy and colleagues suggest five ways in which the validity of a consensus method may be tested.[10] First, the derived consensus can be tested against the 'gold standard', meaning in this context the true answer. For example if a group of individuals are asked questions to which they do not know the answer (but an answer exists), group consensus methods are more likely get closer to the 'truth' than individuals acting alone.[10] In the context of a clinical guideline, where the 'true' or 'correct' way of managing a particular condition is not known, this approach is clearly not helpful.

A second test of validity is the ability of the method to predict the future, i.e. whether a forecast 'came true'. In the case of clinical guidelines, evidence may emerge which either confirms or contradicts the approach recommended in the guideline.

However, this does not mean that the decision made was not the best, given the state of knowledge at the time the guideline was written. Thus, this too is not a helpful test in this context.

A third test is that of 'concurrent validity'. Merrick and colleagues compared the findings of an expert panel with the best evidence available from the current litera-ture, and found them to be almost identical.[24] In the case of guideline development, the reason for using a consensus process is to establish recommendations when there is no available sound evidence to use. Therefore, this would not be an applicable test.

Fourth, the 'internal logic' of the derived consensus can be examined in order to determine the consistency of the decisions (i.e. does one decision fit with the previ-ous and subsequent decisions). The Merrick and Hunter groups both looked at the internal logic of decisions reached by derived consensus and found them to be intern-ally consistent, with only one slight discrepancy.[24,25] This method of testing validity could be applied to clinical guidelines, as recommendations need to follow a logical sequence. Indeed, this is a necessary pre-requisite for the guideline to 'work' and for clinicians to be able to use it.

The measures of validity thus far discussed have looked at whether the derived consensus is intrinsically 'true'. The final approach is to examine outcomes, once the guideline has been put into practice. This indirect measure of validity is clearly the most important because the primary aim of developing a guideline is to improve patient care (with a common secondary aim of reducing costs and making better use of resources). Thus patient morbidity, mortality and satisfaction, professional staff satisfaction and confidence, and costs involved could all be measured before and after a guideline is implemented in order to test its validity.

Very closely linked to the measurement of outcomes is measuring the extent to which a guideline is used, i.e. how influential is it both locally and on a national level. This could also be used as an indirect marker of its validity. In practice, how-ever, the extent to which a guideline is used is more often related to its dissemination and 'marketing' than to its validity (see Chapter 14).

Thus, the only method for assessing the validity of the consensus-based elements within a clinical guideline is to measure the guideline's effect on outcomes. This has been done with several guidelines[26] and it should be done (even if simply by audit) with any implemented guideline.

83

Summary

- Consensus can be used to fill gaps in the evidence chain but should not be used where evidence exists.
- Formal consensus methods are more transparent than informal methods.
- The Delphi process allows a large group of individuals to be involved which may help with implementation later.

References

1. Grimshaw JN, Russell IT. Achieving health gain through clinical guidelines. I: Developing scientifically valid guidelines. Quality in Health Care 1993; 2:243–248.
2. Royal College of Paediatrics and Child Health. Standards for development of clinical guidelines in paediatrics and child health: role of the Royal College of Paediatrics and

Child Health. Report of the quality of practice committee, 2nd edn. London: Royal College of Paediatrics and Child Health; 2001.

3. Thomson R. Construction and use of guidelines. Prescr J 1999; 39:180–187.
4. Armon K, Stephenson TJ, MacFaul R. An evidence and consensus based guideline for the management of a child after a seizure. Emerg Med J 2003; 20:13–20.
5. Harbour R, Miller J. A new system for grading recommendations in evidence based guidelines. BMJ 2001; 323:334–336.
6. Woolf SH. Practice guidelines – a new reality in medicine. II Methods of developing guidelines. Arch Intern Med 1992; 152:946–952.
7. Eccles M, Clapp Z, Grimshaw J et al. North of England evidence based guidelines development project: methods of guideline development. BMJ 1996; 312:760–762.
8. Shekelle PG, Woolf SH, Eccles M, Grimshaw J. Clinical guidelines: developing guidelines. BMJ 1999; 318:593–596.
9. Fletcher SW. Whither scientific deliberation in health policy recommendations? N Engl J Med 1997; 336:1180–1183.
10. Murphy MK, Black NA, Lamping DL et al. Consensus development methods, and their use in clinical guideline development. Health Technol Assess 1998; 2:i–iv, 1–88.
11. Mullen PM. Delphi: myths and reality. J Health Organ Manag 2003; 17(1):37–52.
12. Editorial. The prostate question, unanswered still. Lancet 1997; 349:443.
13. Grimshaw JN, Russell IT. Achieving health gain through clinical guidelines II: Ensuring guidelines change medical practice. Qual Health Care 1994; 3:45–52.
14. Dalkey NC, Helmer O. An experimental application of the Delphi method to the use of experts. Manage Sci 1963; 9:458–467.
15. Pill J. The Delphi method: substance, context, a critique and an annotated bibliography. Socioecon Plann Sci 1971; 5:57–71.
16. Delbecq A, Van de Ven A. A group process model for problem identification and process planning. J Appl Behav Sci 1971; 7:467–492
17. Perry S, Kalberer JTJ. The NIH consensus-development program and the assessment of health-care technologies: the first two years. N Engl J Med 1980; 303:169–172.
18. Cantrill JA, Sibbald B, Buetow S. The Delphi and nominal group techniques in health services research. Int J Pharmacy Pract 1996; 4:67–74.
19. Jones J, Hunter D. Consensus methods for medical and health servises research. BMJ 1995; 311:376–380.
20. Bernstein SJ, Laouri M, Hilbourne LH et al. Coronary angiography: a literature review and ratings of appropriateness and necessity. Vol Report JRA-03. Santa Monica (CA): RAND; 1992.
21. Perry S. The NIH consensus development program, a decade later. N Engl J Med 1987; 317:485–488.
22. Duffield C. The Delphi technique. Aust J Adv Nurs 1988; 6:41–45.
23. Fink A, Kosecoff J, Chassin M, Brook RH. Consensus methods: characteristics and guidelines for use. Am J Public Health 1984; 74:979–983.
24. Merrick NJ, Fink A, Park RE et al. Derivation of clinical indications for carotid endarterectomy by an expert panel. Am J Public Health 1987; 77:187–190.
25. Hunter DJW, McKee CM, Sanderson CFB, Black NA. Appropriate indications for prostatectomy in the UK – results of a consensus panel. J Epidemiol Commun Health 1994; 4:58–64.
26. Armon K, MacFaul R, Hemingway P et al. The impact of presenting problem based guidelines for children with medical problems in an accident and emergency department. Arch Dis Child 2004; 89:159–164.

Chapter 9

The Delphi consensus process

Kate Armon

Aims

- To describe in detail how to set up and run a Delphi process

The Delphi consensus process (also called 'Delphi process', 'Delphi panel', 'Delphi method', or even simply 'Delphi'[1]) is an achievable way of developing formal consensus recommendations in an evidence-based guideline. An overview of the process is given in Figure 9.1.

Defining the rules

It is always easier to understand the rules once you've played the game, so this section will be described later (see Table 9.1). However, it is important to set the rules for each Delphi process at the beginning, so that it remains explicit from the start.

Selecting the panel

Number of participants for a Delphi panel

When combining individual judgements, as in the Delphi approach, more is generally better. When initial opinions are not in agreement, group validity is substantially

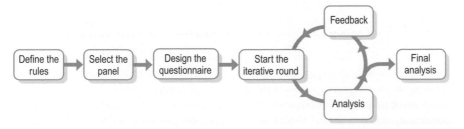

Figure 9.1 Summary of running a Delphi process.

improved with 20 participants rather than 10.[2] A panel which is too large, however, may never reach any consensus. A panel size of between 30 and 50 is manageable.

Example Box 9.1 Selecting a Delphi panel for the guideline 'Seizure – an evidence-based guideline for the management of children presenting post seizure'[3]

- Numbers and types of staff who would be involved in the management of the child presenting with a seizure were estimated.
- The panellists selected were drawn from the United Kingdom, represented practice in both urban and rural settings and were clinicians who would be involved in management of a child after presentation at hospital.
- General practitioners, parents and patients were not included for the Delphi process but these groups were included in other parts of the guideline development.
- Names of individuals were obtained somewhat pragmatically: clinicians were approached who were thought likely to take part! The RCPCH (Royal College of Paediatrics and Child Health) handbook was used to find names and contact details of potential participants.
- Non-paediatric medical personnel and nursing staff were approached after telephoning hospitals and departments for names of enthusiastic clinicians and nurses.

Seventy-seven medical and nursing staff from mixed adult/paediatric A&E departments, paediatric A&E departments, general paediatric departments (both teaching hospital and district general hospital) and specialist paediatric neurology services were invited, of whom 40 agreed to take part.

Final panel make-up:

Staff category	Number
Paediatric trained nurse	2
Mixed adult/paed A&E nurse	2
Paediatric A&E consultant	1
Mixed adult/paed A&E junior	1
Mixed adult/paed A&E consultant	3
DGH consultant paediatrician	15
Junior paediatrician (SHO)	2
Junior paediatrician (SpR)	4
Paediatric neurologist	2
Teaching hospital consultant paediatrician	8
Total	40

Who should be on the panel ('expert' knowledge)?

At the outset, the Delphi technique was used for tapping the knowledge of 'experts'. It is certainly important in the case of guideline development that if the guideline is to gain widespread credibility and acceptability at least some of the members of the panel should be seen to have expert knowledge.

One rather radical definition of 'an expert' is 'anyone who can contribute relevant inputs'.[4] Therefore, in selecting the panel for the Delphi exercise, the primary objective is to obtain the participation of practitioners who are regularly involved with the relevant patients. Clinicians who have a special interest or expertise in the area under consideration should also be enlisted. As most guidelines cross multiple disciplines, each discipline which will use the guideline, or be affected by the use of the guideline, should be represented (see Example Box 9.1). This may include the use of patient representatives as well, although this requires careful consideration when constructing the questionnaire.

Panellists should ideally hold a range of views, such that no particular interests or opinions are allowed to dominate.[5] In choosing the panel, a further factor of fundamental importance is that participants are highly motivated.[6] Thus, when panellists are asked to participate, confidentiality and anonymity and the time that would need to be devoted to it need to be emphasized.

Designing the Delphi questionnaire

Statements

By the final analysis of the process, the Delphi panel will have individually expressed their opinion on a number of statements. The group as a whole will either express agreement with a statement, express disagreement with a statement, or opinion will be evenly split. The statements will often be modified by the panel during the various rounds of the process. However, the first round statements need to be carefully developed by the GDG.

Several methods of developing the statements used in the first Delphi consensus round have been reported in the literature.

- *Literature review.* Statements derived from a review of the literature provided the basis for the earliest Delphi process, using a synthesis of the evidence as it stood. This is still commonly used when dealing with very complex issues.

- *Qualitative round.* This method involves an initial qualitative phase where panellists are asked what they think the important issues are (free expression of opinion). These opinions are then used to generate the statements in the next round. This is particularly useful for deriving a priority list.[7–10]

- *Scenario based.* This involves the use of clinical scenarios (sometimes derived by the panellists themselves) to create statements about what course of action to take in particular situations.[11] This is a useful technique when developing a guideline on symptoms/problems rather than diagnosed conditions.

Whichever method is used, the language of each statement must be clear, so that it is unambiguous. Keep the statements as simple as possible so that the panel only have one aspect of the statement with which to agree or disagree. For example, the statement, 'Children with a Glasgow coma score (GCS) of 8 or less should be intubated and ventilated to protect their airway' can be disagreed in more than one area. Some panellists may disagree with the part of the statement 'GCS score of 8 or less' as the level at which to intubate, while others, who agree with this level of consciousness, may disagree with the need to 'intubate' at this stage and may prefer to support the airway in another way. Two statements may be better in this case to determine when the group agrees with (1) the level of GCS at which airway support is required, and (2) what the appropriate airway support should be at this stage.

It is strongly recommended that the GDG produce draft statements and pilot them on a number of the different groups before initiating round one. Any ambiguity can be identified and statements modified before the Delphi process begins. The process is trying to look for the level of group agreement with the statements, not the level of group comprehension of them!

Background material

How much background material should be provided to the Delphi panel in order for them to understand the issues behind each statement? There are no hard and fast rules here. If a consensus process is required in guideline development, then the evidence base for making a recommendation is not there. It has been suggested that providing the panel with literature to read around the topic engages the panel in the process, making them more likely to respond and complete the rounds.[1] On the other hand, the panelists will be hard-working practitioners, who will not have 5 hours in their schedule to spare to read through 50 articles to help answer one statement.

Others argue that no background material is necessary. Group decisions can be swayed by poor (potentially biased) evidence which is presented to them. As this evidence has already been rejected for not being rigorous enough to provide the evidence base for a recommendation, should it be used to influence the decision of a panel whose opinions are being sought for their own validity? Decision-making can be biased in a number of ways when reviewing literature.[12] By providing no background material the participants' views can potentially be sought 'fresh' without any influence from the GDG.

Whatever background material is provided, the GDG must try to engage the panel while not biasing their decisions. Ensure that a record of what is sent out with the statements is kept so that the process remains transparent.

Panellists' responses

The panellists need to be able to indicate how they agree with a statement. Various methods can be employed. One Delphi panel was asked to determine whether, in given situations, certain procedures were 'Necessary' (i.e. crucial to the patient's management), 'Appropriate' or 'Inappropriate'.[13] Another Delphi panel made up of surgeons were asked to predict the percentage of procedures that could be carried out as a day case, and then rate the confidence with which they held this view on a five-point scale.[14] This refinement of asking for the participants' 'confidence' in a statement allows the participants to express uncertainty or partial agreement.[11]

A 9-point Likert scale[15] is a practical way of giving panellists the ability to express different levels of agreement, and can be relatively easily analysed statistically (see Example Box 9.2).

Starting the rounds

Once the questionnaire is designed, the first round can begin. All the panellists will have to have instructions on how to respond to the statements, the background material, a timescale for responding and some means of returning the forms.

For subsequent rounds, the analysis and feedback will also be needed to allow the panellists to re-think their original level of agreement in the light of the whole group's response.

The amount of paper can build up (see Example Box 9.3). Delphi panels can be coordinated electronically, to reduce costs and save trees!

Example Box 9.2 Use of a Likert scale for expressing agreement for the evidence-based guideline 'The management of reduced consciousness in children'16

Statement 5

'Children with a Glasgow coma score of 8 or less should be intubated and ventilated to protect their airway.'

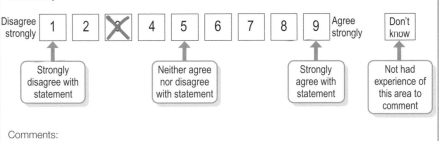

Comments:

Example Box 9.3 Organizing the Delphi process for the guideline 'Diarrhoea and vomiting – an evidence-based guideline for children presenting with diarrhoea with or without vomiting'17

Pilot

A first round Delphi pack was piloted on five staff: two consultants, two trainee paediatricians and a nurse specialist. The pack was then revised where necessary to improve clarity and remove ambiguity.

First round

The following components of the pack were indexed and bound in a large file and sent by post to each panellist:

Instructions	An introductory letter
	• The panellists were asked to read the literature review, referring to papers if they wished, and to rate their level of agreement with each statement as written.
	• They were encouraged to make free text comments on the questionnaire whenever they wished.
Background material	The literature review
	The critical appraisal abstraction sheets for all articles cited (with strength and grading of evidence)
	A copy of all articles cited
Questionnaire	35 statements to respond to
	A response form detailing each statement with a 1–9 Likert scale and space for comments
Reply	A stamped addressed envelope for response form returns

A reminder letter was sent and a subsequent telephone call was made to non-responders if the statements had not been returned after 4 weeks.

Second round

All panellists received by post:

Instructions	Letter of thanks and instructions
Background material	Discussion document including the first round analysis and further literature review
	The papers and critical appraisal for new literature

Continued

Example Box 9.3 *Continued*

Questionnaire	20 statements (statements which were agreed upon by consensus in the previous round were not included in subsequent rounds)
	Response form with remaining statements and Likert scale as before

Third round
All panellists received by post as above for the second round, with the remaining statements that had not yet achieved consensus.

Final analysis
After three rounds.

Analysis of responses

A quantitative analysis of the responses is a key feature of the Delphi method. How the analysis is performed is highly dependent upon the format used to record the panellists' responses. If a Likert scale is used, the responses can be numerically summarized relatively easily (see Example Box 9.4).

Example Box 9.4 Numerical analysis of responses from a Delphi process statement for the guideline 'Seizure – an evidence-based guideline for the management of children presenting post seizure'[3]

Statement 15
'A child who has had a simple febrile convulsion, where no source of infection has been found clinically, should have a urine sample (clean catch, suprapubic aspirate or catheter sample) taken for microscopy and culture'.

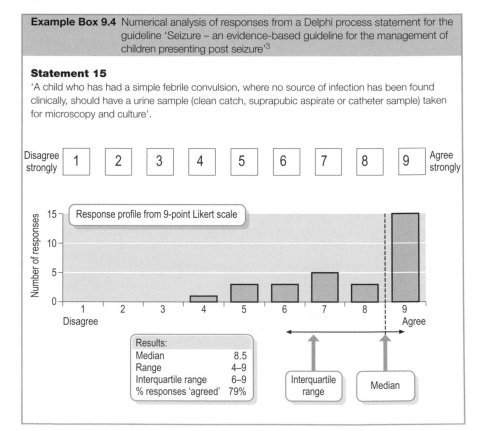

Definition of consensus

The definition of consensus is clearly crucial to the whole consensus development process, and it is essential that it be decided before the process starts. Again there is no right answer and several definitions of consensus have been used in different Delphi processes.[18] Usually, consensus is accepted when 75% or more of participants agree. If greater than 25% disagree there is lack of consensus.

On the 9-point Likert scale as in Example Box 9.2, responses in boxes 7, 8 or 9 can be grouped as agreeing with the statement. Responses in boxes 1, 2 or 3 can be grouped as disagreeing with the statement. Responses in boxes 4, 5 or 6 can be grouped as neither agreeing nor disagreeing with the statement – group 'ambivalence'. Therefore, if 75% of the responses are grouped in the 7, 8 or 9 boxes, this could be the definition of consensus agreement chosen by the GDG before the Delphi process begins.

There is further discussion in the literature about the exclusion of 'outliers' – those expressing an extreme view. Some researchers exclude extreme views prior to reporting the percentage agreement (see Example Box 9.5).

Example Box 9.5	Definition of consensus for 'Seizure – an evidence-based guideline for the management of children presenting post seizure'3
Response format	9 point Likert scale (1 = Strongly disagree; 9 = Strongly agree)
Analysis	Calculate median response Remove outliers (one sixth of the responses furthest from the median) Review the remaining responses
Definition of agreement with a statement	Remaining responses (83% – a stricter definition than the standard 75%) must **all** lie within the 3-point range 6–8 or 7–9
Definition of disagreement with a statement	Remaining responses (83%) must **all** lie within the 3-point range 1–3 or 2–4
Definition of ambivalence to the statement	Remaining responses (83%) must **all** lie within the 3-point range 3–5, 4–6 or 5–7
Definition of no consensus within the group	Remaining responses are distributed with at least one eighth (12.5%) in boxes 1–3 **and** at least one eighth (12.5%) in boxes 7–9

Feedback	• Statements with clear agreement were included in the guideline recommendations and removed from subsequent rounds.
	• Statements not reaching consensus were either
	  ◦ removed from the guideline if the comments suggested a fundamental difference of opinion or
	  ◦ modified to clarify points raised by the Delphi panel and included in the next round.
	• Statements rated with ambivalence by the panel were modified and included in the next round.

Feedback

Quantitative

There is limited information on numerical feedback in the literature. It is, however, generally acknowledged that the use of the median and interquartile range is probably the most useful method to feed back the range of views from previous rounds.[2,5,7,19] Alternatively you can show the number of participants making each choice within each box of the Likert scale (see Example Box 9.4).

Qualitative

Feedback of the panel's comments is useful for several reasons. First, it allows the panellists' second choices to be based on informational feedback rather than simply normative feedback. Second, participants feel that their opinion is more valued if their comments are taken into account. Comments can be grouped together into themes and summarized or left unchanged. Remember, all comments need to be kept anonymous (but the GDG need to record who made which comment, so the process can be reviewed later).

Modifying statements

- It is simplest to remove any statements that achieve consensus agreement from subsequent rounds, so that the rounds become shorter and simpler for participants.

- Those statements which achieve 'near' consensus can be left unchanged allowing the panel to modify their responses based solely on the numerical feedback of the group response.

- When consensus is not achieved by a significant margin look at the comments made by the panel. If there is ambiguity in the statement, or the panellists suggest a re-wording of the statement, this will be obvious from the comments. The statement can be modified in the light of these responses (see Example Box 9.6).

- If consensus has not been achieved because of a true difference in opinion, it is unlikely that agreement will be reached. The statement should be removed from subsequent rounds. However, this is important information for developing the guideline's recommendations. Not only is there no evidence to make a recommendation in this area, but a panel of practitioners cannot agree on a course of action either. The guideline document should reflect this and recommend that local practice preferences should be looked into during the implementation of the guideline. This will clearly need to be highlighted as an area of high priority for research in the future.

Along with the quantitative and qualitative feedback, the modified statements can be complemented with further background material in the subsequent rounds if needed.

Example Box 9.6 Modifying statements in subsequent rounds of the Delphi process for the guideline 'Seizure – an evidence-based guideline for the management of children presenting post seizure'[3]

Clinical question	In a child with a simple febrile seizure, who does not have serious features on examination, but who has been treated with oral antibiotics, is there an increased risk of meningitis?
Statements Round 1	(a) Those children with a simple febrile seizure who have had prior antibiotic treatment should have a lumbar puncture (LP) performed. (b) If an LP is not performed in a child with a simple febrile convulsion and prior antibiotic treatment, the child should be admitted and observed.
Results	(a) Definition of 'ambivalence' between panellists met. Median 6, min 2, max 8, interquartile range 4–7. (b) Definition of 'ambivalence' met. Median 7, min 4, max 9, interquartile range 6–8.
Comments	(a) Rather say 'strongly consider' an LP than 'should have'(n = 5). If well, clinical observation is sufficient (n = 9). If clear clinical reason for antibiotics, other than meningitis, then this can be accepted as cause of fever and no LP performed (n = 3). (b) Only need admission if clinically suspicious; community follow-up should be sufficient (n = 4). Depends on duration and indication for antibiotics (n = 1).
Statements Round 2	Those children with a simple febrile seizure, >1 year of age and with no serious historical or examination findings indicating meningitis who have had prior antibiotic treatment: (c) Should be admitted to an acute paediatric facility for a period of observation (at least 2 hours). (d) Should have an LP performed. (e) Do not require admission if the source of bacterial infection is still evident and this does not require hospital treatment.
Results	(c) Definition of 'agreement' met. All responses in boxes 7–9 (after removal of outliers). (d) Definition of 'disagreement' between panellists met. Median 5, min 3, max 7, interquartile range 4–6. (e) Definition of 'ambivalence' between panellists met. Median 6, min 3, max 9, interquartile range 4–8.
Comments	(c) May not need admission (n = 2). (d) Depends on source of fever and indication for antibiotics (n = 2). Depends on clinical picture and focus of fever (n = 2). (e) Depends on parental view, and whether temperature can be controlled at home (n = 3). Over-diagnosis of otitis media may influence this (n = 2).
Final analysis	Statement 'c' incorporated into the guideline recommendations (Grade D).

93

Final analysis

When to stop the Delphi process is another issue which is not strictly defined. In terms of the 'pure' Delphi methodology, the process should be stopped when 'stability' is reached (i.e. no statistical change in the levels of agreement between rounds or when consensus has been achieved). For practical guideline developers it is reasonable to decide on a pre-defined number of rounds (often two or three).

Defining the rules (at last!)

So now you know how the process works, it is important to define the rules of play right at the beginning (Table 9.1). These should be documented to keep the process explicit and open to review later.

Incorporating patients in the consensus process

When selecting a Delphi panel, all the stakeholders should be included. Patients are a significant stakeholder in the guideline and should be considered for inclusion in the Delphi process. The difficulty with including patients on a multidisciplinary panel will be their lack of knowledge in the many fields of medicine, which are likely to be covered by the process.

Two possible solutions have been suggested:

1. Select them along with a multidisciplinary expert panel, but ensure that there are specific statements which seek patient preferences to involve them in the process.

Table 9.1 Defining the rules of a Delphi process

Selecting the panel	How many panellists? Which specialties?

Questionnaire	Will there be a qualitative round to help determine statements?
	What should the background material comprise?
	In which format will responses be made?
	    (e.g. Likert scale, Yes/No answers)
	If the topic of the Delphi is broad, will a 'Don't know' option be required
	    so panellists without experience in a particular field don't guess at a
	    response?
	What is the time limit for responses to be returned?
	What is an acceptable number of responders?

Analysis	How will the responses be analysed? How will outliers be handled? How will consensus be defined?
Feedback	How will comments be fed back to panellists? When will modifications be made to the statements and when will they be fed back unchanged?
Rounds	How many rounds will the process take?

Having a 'Don't know' box next to the Likert scale will hopefully prevent panellists (including the patient representatives) from guessing the 'right' answer, if they have no experience in that field.

2. Use a separate patient Delphi panel to help determine patient views. This process can also be used to produce patient information leaflets – the information which is important for the patients to know is possibly best decided by them.

Summary

- An achievable formal consensus methodology for most guideline developers to use.
- Define the rules at the beginning.
- Incorporate as many stakeholder groups as possible.

References

1. Mullen PM. Delphi: myths and reality. J Health Organ Manag 2003; 17(1):37–52.
2. Murphy MK, Black NA, Lamping DL et al. Consensus development methods, and their use in clinical guideline development. Health Technol Assess 1998; 2:i–iv, 1–88.
3. Armon K, Stephenson TJ, MacFaul R et al. An evidence and consensus based guideline for the management of a child after a seizure. Emerg Med J 2003; 20:13–20.
4. Pill J. The Delphi method: substance, context, a critique and an annotated bibliography. Socioecon Plann Sci 1971; 5:57–71.
5. Jones J, Hunter D. Consensus methods for medical and health services research. BMJ 1995; 311:376–380.
6. Duffield C. The Delphi technique. Aust J Adv Nurs 1988; 6:41–45.
7. Charlton JRH, Patrick DL, Matthews G, West PA. Spending priorities in Kent: a Delphi study. J Epidemiol Commun Health 1981; 35:288–292.
8. Gabbay J, Francis L. How much day surgery? Delphic predictions. BMJ 1988; 297:1249–1252.
9. Harrington JM. Research priorities in occupational medicine: a survey of United Kingdom medical opinion by the Delphi technique. Occup Environ Med 1994; 51:289–294.
10. Jones J, Sanderson C, Black N. What will happen to the quality of care with fewer junior doctors? A Delphi study of consultant physicians' views. J R Coll Physicians Lond 1992; 26:36–40.
11. Koplan JP, Farer LS. Choice of preventive treatment for isoniazid-resistant tuberculous infection. JAMA 1980; 244:2736–2740.
12. Kaptchuk T. Effect of interpretive bias on research evidence. BMJ 2003; 326:1453–1455.
13. Kahan JP, Bernstein SJ, Leape LL et al. Measuring the necessity of medical procedures. Med Care 1994; 32:357–365.
14. Grainger C, Griffiths R. Day surgery – how much is possible? A Delphi consensus among surgeons. Public Health 1994; 108:257–266.
15. Barnett, V. Sample survey principles and methods. London: Hodder; 1991.

16. The Paediatric Accident and Emergency Research Group. The mangement of a child with a decreased conscious level. 2005. www.nottingham.ac.uk/paediatric-guideline
17. Armon K, Stephenson TJ, MacFaul R et al. An evidence and consensus based guideline for acute diarrhoea management. Arch Dis Child 2001; 85:132–142.
18. Fink A, Kosecoff J, Chassin M, Brook RH. Consensus methods: characteristics and guidelines for use. Am J Public Health 1984; 74:979–983.
19. Dalkey NC, Helmer O. An experimental application of the Delphi method to the use of experts. Manage Sci 1963; 9:458–467.

Health economics

Hannah-Rose Douglas

Aims

- To describe how and when to incorporate economic analysis into guideline development
- To briefly describe types of economic analysis used in guidelines
- To describe the resources used by the health economist

Health economics is concerned with healthcare resources, scarcity and choice.[1] It aims to improve the health of the population through the efficient use of resources. Therefore, it applies to every clinical decision.

Health economic evaluation is *not* about *costs*, but about *cost-effectiveness*. The most expensive treatment will not be outlawed if it is the most effective for that condition and releases resources for use elsewhere. Similarly the cheapest treatment will not be hailed champion automatically if it provides little benefit to the patient. Therefore, evidence of the effectiveness of an intervention is just as important to the health economist as the cost.

Clinical guidelines developed at a national level will not usually be resourced to the extent of employing health economists for the full length of the guideline development process. Therefore, it is important for those producing the guidelines to have some practical understanding of:

- the principles and practice – both good and bad – of economic evaluation;
- what is feasible in terms of incorporating economic evaluation into guidelines; and
- what practical steps they need to take to get the economic evidence for consideration.

How to incorporate health economics into guideline recommendations

Economic considerations should be a part of every recommendation which the guideline produces (Figure 10.1). This does not mean that for every recommendation

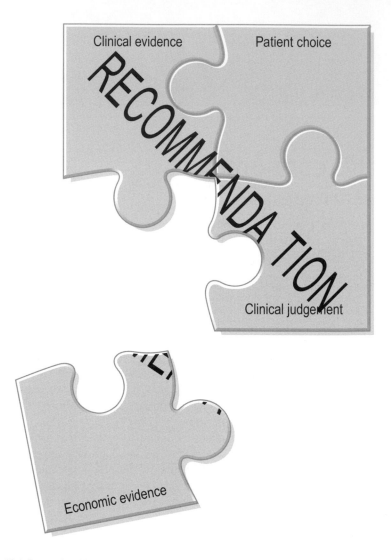

Figure 10.1 Economic evidence forms part of the jigsaw of forming recommendations.

a detailed economic evaluation of the topic needs to be completed. It means that consideration has to be given to both the clinical effectiveness and the cost together of implementing a recommendation by healthcare providers. Both research evidence and clinical experience can be brought to bear on these issues.

Options for incorporating health economics into guideline recommendations

■ Discussing cost-effectiveness issues at GDG meetings and documenting the likely costs alongside the effectiveness of an intervention in the guideline documentation;

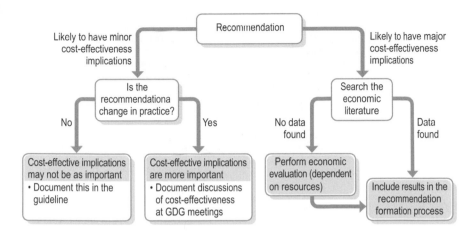

Figure 10.2 Algorithm for incorporating health economic considerations into guidelines.

- Documenting whether a recommendation is a change to current practice, no change to current practice or will improve adherence to best practice, as these will have different implications in terms of cost-effectiveness;
- Searching the economic literature for data to be included in the guideline;
- Performing a formal cost-effectiveness analysis.

The GDG need to decide early on where the contentious cost-effectiveness issues will be in the guideline. They should focus their attention on a couple of key areas where cost is perceived to be a significant hurdle to implementation of a recommendation (Figure 10.2).

When to use formal economic evaluations

An economic evaluation compares the costs and outcomes (both benefits and harms) of competing healthcare interventions. A full economic evaluation is a major under taking. However, there are many instances in a guideline where this is not necessary:

- where two or more alternatives have exactly the same outcome but one is cheaper – the cheapest one should be recommended (freeing up healthcare resources for use elsewhere) – e.g. reducing fever using paracetamol or ibuprofen: both are equally effective but paracetamol is cheaper over-the-counter.
- where two or more alternatives have the same cost but one is more effective – the most effective should be recommended (producing more health benefits overall for the same cost) – e.g. the cost of a long-acting methylphenidate for attention-deficit hyperactivity disorder is the same as that of a shorter-acting one but is more effective in keeping a child attentive in lessons.

The 'cost-effectiveness plane' (Figure 10.3) shows where economic evaluation is warranted and where it is not.

Using Figure 10.3, clearly intervention A should be recommended over intervention B, and intervention E should be recommended over intervention A. The areas where the waters are muddy need further examination.

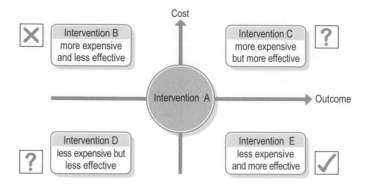

Figure 10.3 The 'cost-effectiveness plane'.

Table 10.1

Types of economic evaluation

Method of economic evaluation	Healthcare resources measured in	Outcomes measured
Cost-utility analysis	Monetary units (£)	Quality-adjusted life years
Cost-effectiveness analysis	Monetary units (£)	Natural units, e.g. life years saved, acute episodes averted
Cost-benefit analysis	Monetary units (£)	Monetary units (£)
Cost analysis	Monetary units (£)	None

- Intervention C costs more but has a better outcome. Is the better outcome 'worth' the extra cost?
- Intervention D costs less but has a smaller benefit. Is the reduction in outcome acceptable to save money to be spent elsewhere on health needs?

The decisions about recommending interventions C or D should be made by weighing up the expected benefits and costs of health care but this is rarely done *explicitly*. People use 'intuition', and base their decisions on 'what has always been done' or on political expediency or 'cost pressures' (that is, what someone else thinks is a good use of healthcare resources). Only in a few areas do decision-makers make their criteria for choosing how to use scarce resources explicit. Guideline developers are being encouraged to make explicit economic considerations when making recommendations, partly due to government bodies such as the National Institute for Health and Clinical Excellence (NICE) that use economic evaluation in this way.

Which types of economic analysis can be used in clinical guidelines?

Economic evaluations can be used as a tool for making recommendations more transparent and sometimes more defendable. However their applications and limitations need to be clearly understood in order for them to be useful.

There are many different types of economic evaluation of health care. The differences depend mainly on how the health outcome is measured (Table 10.1).

Cost-utility analysis has been used to standardize the comparison between different outcome measures. If a study finds that you need to treat 5000 patients with aspirin to prevent one stroke, how does that compare with another study which finds that you need to treat 300 patients with a statin to prevent one myocardial infarction. What is the different level of morbidity associated with the different diseases? Also when assessing two or more possible treatments, both quality of life and mortality outcomes (quantity of life) are important, but how do they compare?

The aim of a cost-utility analysis is to turn all health outcomes into commensurable units of health, combining both quantity and quality of life into one unit of outcome (see Example Box 10.1).

In theory, this approach ensures that all healthcare interventions can be evaluated on a level playing field by comparing all interventions in the same units of outcome (preferably a QALY – quality-adjusted life year). If we knew society's maximum willingness to pay for an additional QALY then we would have a criterion for deciding whether an intervention was cost-effective, i.e. the cost per QALY was less than society's maximum willingness to pay for a QALY (say £20 000 per QALY). If we were comparing two or more alternatives, we could calculate the additional cost per QALY of a recommendation to switch from one to another, and assess whether that lay within our £20 000 per QALY cut-off for cost-effectiveness.

Example Box 10.1 QALYs

A *quality-adjusted life year* is a measure of the benefit of a medical treatment. It is based on the number of years of life that would be added by receiving the treatment. Each year in perfect health is assigned the value of 1. If the extra years would not be lived in full health, for example if the patient would lose a limb, or be blind or be confined to a wheelchair, then the extra life years are given a value between 0 (the value for death) and 1 to account for this.

Calculating QALYs
Quality-adjusted life years are calculated in two stages.

The first stage is to describe a disease in terms of a specific *health state*. Quality of life instruments such as the EuroQol[2] have been designed to allow every imaginable health state to be described in terms of simple descriptions of the impact on an individual's ability to live a full life. All states of health from those close to death (or worse than death) to perfect health can be described in a combination of these levels.

Time in years in these health states is then multiplied by this quality of life weight to give a composite score. Actuarial life expectancy figures are required for this as well (e.g. saving the life of a 1-year-old child with intensive care treatment and return to full health compared with the same treatment provided to an 80-year-old will have different QALYs due to life expectancy).

All QALYs are assumed to be perfectly divisible, and an individual is assumed to be indifferent between quality and quantity of life, which means they are equally happy with 4 additional years in perfect health or 8 years in a health state with a weight of 0.50.

The logic is clear and defendable. The practice, however, is far from straightforward. There are methodological challenges in measuring outcomes in this way, all of which are recognized and well understood by the health economic community.

Progress has been made in research to collect robust population-based data on the impact of different health states on quality of life in order to derive robust quality of life weightings for a wide range of health states. It is important, therefore, that those reviewing economic evaluation evidence ensure that this research is based on the best available UK population-based evidence to derive QALY estimates. The cost-utility approach is now seen by many as the optimal method of economic evaluation in the UK.

Incremental cost-effectiveness ratio or ICER is the standard way of presenting health economic results. Incremental cost-effectiveness ratios show the additional cost per unit of outcome of one intervention (say a new operation, or newly recommended medicine) over another (either an older technology, or 'usual practice') (see Example Box 10.2 for an example of deriving an ICER).

Example Box 10.2 How to calculate an incremental cost-effectiveness ratio

Consider two alternative procedures for the same life-threatening condition, such as cancer. In a cohort of 1000 people with the disease Treatment A prevents 120 premature deaths. Procedure B prevents 180 premature deaths. A costs £2500 per person. B costs £4900 per person.

	Total cost	Total benefit (lives saved)	Incremental cost	Incremental effectiveness	ICER
Procedure A	£2.5 million	120			
Procedure B	£4.9 million	180	£2.4 million	60 lives saved	£40000 per life saved

---

An ICER can be expressed in any unit of outcome, such as lives saved, or in QALYs.

$$\frac{£ \text{ cost of intervention A} - £ \text{ cost of intervention B}}{QALY \text{ for intervention A} - QALY \text{ for intervention B}}$$

Cost-effectiveness analysis is very common as this can be an add-on to clinical studies of efficacy, such as RCTs, using the same units of outcome for the analysis. The limitations are that the results do not really help in deciding whether a health outcome is worth the additional cost as the units measured are highly specific. No straightforward comparison can be made for the best use of the health budget from cost-effectiveness data. For example, is the aversion of an acute episode of schizophrenia 'worth' the additional cost of the mental health programme designed to do this? Is the cost of saving a fatal car accident 'worth' the cost of road humps? If you have to decide to implement one new healthcare initiative, how can you compare like for like with such different outcome data?

Cost-benefit analysis is almost never performed in healthcare evaluation because of the problems of translating health outcomes into monetary units. It is far more common in transport or environmental economic evaluation.

Cost analysis provides information on the cost of an intervention or a health service. This is not helpful on its own in making decisions about whether an intervention is worth implementing. It can provide information on the *affordability* of an intervention to a health service. But affordability is a separate question from whether an intervention is cost-effective, that is, whether the health benefits are worth the costs. In order to make recommendations in a clinical guideline, cost-effectiveness – *not* cost analysis – is the information that is required.

What can realistically be achieved in a clinical guideline?

The way that cost-effectiveness analysis can be incorporated in a clinical guideline will depend on whether the resources are available to employ a health economist to focus on this aspect of its development. The input of a health economist is useful because they approach the specific questions addressed in the guideline from a different angle. Put very simply, the clinician may ask of a healthcare intervention, 'Does it work?'. A health economist will ask, 'Should we do it?'. To answer the second question, information on both the outcomes and the resources used are needed.

If a qualified health economist is required but there is no extra funding in the guideline development budget for this, ask a health economist to be part of the GDG at the start of the process. As all GDG members volunteer their services, being involved from the start may encourage the health economist to work for free also! Try your local medical school for contacts. Asking a health economist to provide an economic evaluation at the end of the guideline development process without input ('ownership') from the start may be a far less attractive option to them, reducing the likelihood that they will collaborate.

However, there are ways of incorporating health economic concepts into a clinical guideline without the need for a trained health economist. The group developing the clinical guideline can incorporate health economics in the following ways:

Agreeing where cost-effectiveness needs to be formally considered and where it does not

The guideline group should highlight the specific topics where strong health economic arguments are needed in the guideline (see Figure 10.2). In every case where a recommendation is considered a change in current practice or where a recommendation may not be implemented because of affordability concerns, the cost-effectiveness judgements should be clearly documented.

Reviewing the published literature

Like published clinical evidence, the quality of cost-effectiveness evidence can be highly variable, especially older studies. Studies can be appraised against a standardized checklist.[3] However, there are specific sources of health economic data that are more reliable:

- The Health Technology Assessment Programme is a good source of economic analysis.[4]

- NICE technology appraisals.[5]
- The National Health Service Economic Evaluation Database (NHSEED)[6] and the Health Economic Evaluations Database (HEED)[7] provide excellent commentaries on published economic evaluations that can be a guide to whether the results of the studies can be used to support making recommendations in a clinical guideline.

Considering the cost-effectiveness of recommendations

In many cases, there will be an absence of high-quality cost-effectiveness evidence to support recommendations. In these situations, where recommendations are made, it is good practice to provide the rationale on which the decision has been made. This level of explicitness will increase the transparency of the reasoning behind the recommendation and allow others to challenge your reasoning if they do not agree.

In every section of a clinical guideline where NHS resources are being used, the guideline could consider:

- What are the benefits?
- What are the risks/harms?
- How did the guideline group weigh up the benefits/risks and costs to come to their decision?

The important thing is to demonstrate that the guideline group has thought about the resource implications of any changes from the status quo.

There are many ways to go about this, but perhaps one way would be to consider the following:

A recommendation that there is no change in current practice

Be explicit about why you believe NHS resources are well spent on this intervention (e.g. investigation or treatment) and on what evidence the judgements are based.

A recommendation that should lead to better adherence to good practice

Say what the likely resource consequences are, e.g. more referrals to secondary care, but more effective use of specialist care, so better use of expensive specialist services.

A recommendation that there is a change in practice

Document clearly the discussions and outcomes around cost issues (e.g. 'the GDG consensus was that this would be a good use of resources because…' or 'this would free up resources because…').

Where to find health economic data

If you want to perform a cost-utility or cost-effectiveness analysis you will need a health economist to perform the analysis. The guideline development group may need to provide some of the data which will be used in the calculations. Some of

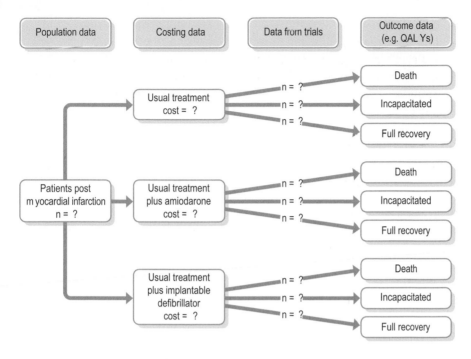

Figure 10.4 A clinical decision tree for implantable defibrillators in patients post myocardial infarction and what data may be needed to perform a cost-utility analysis.

the factors and data sources which are used in cost-utility analysis are explained below:

- *A clinical decision tree* (see Figure 10.4). This is a diagram which demonstrates the possible treatment options for a specific condition and the probabilities associated with all the possible outcomes. This can be drawn up with help from the GDG. Data regarding the number of patients with the condition who have a good outcome with treatment A and a good outcome with treatment B can be found from epidemiology studies and RCTs of the treatments.

- *Population data.* Use epidemiological studies to get an idea of the frequency of the disease in the population concerned. Hospital event statistics can also be used but provide very crude data. www.hesonline.nhs.uk

- *Costing data.* Think about the treatment and staffing costs.
  - *NHS national tariffs.* These were first introduced in the NHS in 2005/6. They are the prices paid to NHS providers for all clinical procedures, based on NHS reference costs for the previous year. www.dh.gov.uk/PolicyAndGuidance/OrganisationPolicy/FinanceAndPlanning/NHSReferenceCosts/fs/en. Click on 'Payment by results' and follow the link to national tariffs for the current year.
  - *Electronic drug tariff.* The current price paid for drugs and appliances supplied against an NHS presciption by dispensing pharmacists. www.ppa.org.uk/ppa/edt_intro.htm

- *Personal and social services.* Costs (not the same as price paid to suppliers of these services) of NHS and social service staff and services (e.g. cost of a GP consultation, cost per session of local authority day care). www.pssru.ac.uk/

■ *Data from trials.* RCTs and systematic reviews of the intervention in question will provide the numbers surviving in good health or not in both treatment and control groups. Cohort studies may help with prognosis in control groups also.

■ *Outcome data.* The ideal measure is the QALY. There are lists of QALYs for various health states available:

- The Health Outcomes Data Repository (HoDAR) based at the Cardiff Research Consortium (www.crc-limited.co.uk) has clinical outcomes data including QALY values for a very wide range of diseases that researchers can subscribe to (at a cost).

- NICE Technology Appraisals also present outcome data in QALYs. Their reports are a good source of data on QALY values for a range of diseases.

A formal cost-effectiveness or cost-utility analysis requires the input of an experienced health economist.

Summary

- All recommendations have cost-effectiveness implications; therefore think like an economist and ask not just 'Does it work?' but 'Should we do it?'
- Be explicit about how the economic judgements have been made in the decision-making processes.
- Good-quality economic evaluation is very difficult. Select an area where implementation may be inhibited by affordability considerations to make the case for a health economist to undertake a formal economic evaluation.

Further reading

Office of Health Economics
A very straightforward introduction for school students and others who want to understand health economic concepts. www.oheschools.org/ohe.pdf

Bandolier series
For a one-page summary of concepts used in health economic evaluation:
What is a QALY? www.jr2.ox.ac.uk/bandolier/band24/b24-7.html
Using QALYs in decision-making. www.jr2.ox.ac.uk/bandolier/band62/b62-8.html
Economics and health care. www.jr2.ox.ac.uk/bandolier/band18/b18-4.html

Evidence-based medicine
Series of slightly longer articles, going through explanations and worked examples, such as 'Implementing QALYs', which shows the steps taken to arrive at a cost per QALY.
www.evidence-based-medicine.co.uk/What_is_series.html

National Health and Research Council, Australia
'How to compare the costs and benefits: evaluation of economic evidence' – a very detailed description of incorporating cost-effectiveness analysis into national guidelines.
www.nhmrc.gov.au/publications/synopses/cp73syn.htm

References

1. Eccles M, Mason J. How to develop cost-conscious guidelines. Health Technol Assess 2001; 5(16):1–69.
2. EQ-5D – An instrument to describe and value health. www.euroqol.org
3. Drummond M, Jefferson T. Guidelines for authors and peer reviewers of economic submissions to the BMJ. BMJ 1996; 331:275–283.
4. The NHS Health Technology Assessment Programme. www.ncchta.org
5. NICE technology appraisals. www.nice.org.uk
6. Centre for Reviews and Dissemination. NHS Economic Evaluation Database. www.york.ac.uk/inst/crd/crddatabases.htm
7. Health Economic Evaluations Database. www.ohe-heed.com

References

[illegible]

Chapter 11

Making recommendations

Monica Lakhanpaul

Aims

- To describe briefly the components required for forming recommendations
- To highlight the importance of clinical judgement throughout this process
- To explain how to make the recommendation-forming process transparent
- To discuss the pros and cons of different grading systems

Having spent a vast amount of time and resources gathering individual papers, assessing them for their methodological quality, degree of bias and, in turn, grading them using whichever grading system has been chosen, the highlight of the guideline process arrives. It is time to make the recommendations.

Why are recommendations important?

1. They decrease variation and standardize the care across the country.
2. They bring clinical care in line with current evidence and good practice.
3. They change practice to reduce inappropriate interventions or treatments.
4. They make the most efficient use of economic resources in relation to health outcomes.
5. *They may be the only part of the guideline that is read!*

Why are recommendations so difficult to make?

Because making recommendations is an art, not a precise science!

Ingredients required to make a recommendation

A recommendation is not a direct quote from a research paper. In fact a recommendation is often several steps removed from the evidence. This is because of the various

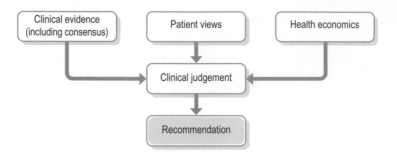

Figure 11.1 Components required for recommendation formation.

pieces of additional information which are added into the process (Figure 11.1) and the clinical judgement required to make sense of it all.

Clinical judgement and its role in guidelines

Organizations such as the Scottish Intercollegiate Guidelines Network[1], the National Health and Medical Research Council,[2] the Royal College of Paediatrics and Child Health,[3] the National Health Service Executive[4] and the National Institute of Health and Clinical Excellence[5] have developed guidance on the methodology required to produce high-quality guidelines.

One could ask why a highly qualified technical team could not develop a guideline without input from clinicians? This would reduce any bias offered by clinicians who have their own interests at heart and sometimes have views counter to that of the evidence. However, the guideline might not be as practical or achievable as one developed with input from the 'troops on the ground'.

Clinical practice needs to be kept up to date with current evidence but we must realize that evidence is not applicable to all patients. It is clear that healthcare professionals need to use *both* clinical expertise and best available evidence to make appropriate decisions.[6]

Some examples of why data extracted from the literature cannot be directly converted into a recommendation are provided below:

1. The population studied may be too small to generalize the data to a larger population or may not relate to the population in question in the guideline.

Example Box 11.1

Clinical question:
In patients with diabetes and hypertension should drug A (e.g. a long-acting dihydropyridine calcium-channel blocker) be used over drug B (e.g. a beta-blocker) to prevent stroke?

Literature:
Drug A is better than drug B to prevent strokes in hypertensive patients. Diabetic patients, however, were excluded from all the trials.

Continued

> **Example Box 11.1** *Continued*
>
> **Judgement:**
> Even though drug A is a better drug to prevent stroke in general, does this still apply to the population with diabetes? Are there any other factors that need to be taken into consideration when deciding whether this treatment is useful in this particular population?

2. The included age range of the study may not be applicable to the population that you want to apply the guideline to. Literature may describe an age range from 0 to 15 years but only two of the patients included may have been under the age of 1 year. Therefore a judgement needs to be made about how applicable the data are to this group of patients.

> **Example Box 11.2**
>
> **Clinical question:**
> Are chest X-rays required for the assessment of pneumonia in children with respiratory distress?
>
> **Literature:**
> Chest X-rays do not affect the management of children with respiratory distress and clinical signs of pneumonia. However, only three children under the age of 1 year have been included in the studies and no children under 6 months were included.
>
> **Judgement:**
> Should the recommendation apply to all children or to a subgroup of children?
>
> **Final recommendation:**
> Children over the age of 1 year do not require a chest X-ray for the assessment of pneumonia.

3. The literature does not answer the clinical question that you really want to ask, i.e. are the questions answered by the literature the same as those being asked by the guideline?

4. Due to health economics, the inclusion of a recommendation in a guideline cannot be justified. Following a literature review it may be obvious that one treatment or intervention or diagnostic test is better than another but the question then has to be asked how much better is A than B. How much of a difference will it make to a patient's survival or quality of life? Can the cost of the new intervention (if more than the old one) be justified, since increasing the costs in one area means movement of money from another?

Incorporating the experiences of clinical practice into a recommendation may make it applicable to other patient groups rather than just the populations covered by the studies.

Incorporating the realities of clinical decision-making into recommendations makes for easier implementation by other clinicians. If no-one asks whether it is workable to implement a recommendation into everyday practice, then the recommendation may become an aspiration rather than a reality.

The most important consideration to be made is whether it is of more benefit than harm to the patients for the recommendation to be implemented.

For all of the reasons given above, a technical team alone may not make a usable clinical guideline.

Making the transparent leap from evidence to recommendation

A guideline recommendation is like an onion. If you look at it on the surface it should be very simple. As you learn more about it you realize that it needs to be unravelled to find the original evidence that it was based on.

Some critics of guidelines misunderstand that recommendations are not a direct transcription of the evidence from the literature and this needs to be addressed. If left ignored then this has the potential to produce a lot of difficulties during the implementation of the guideline. Be aware of your critics and reduce their chances to criticize the recommendations by being explicit about what happened (Figure 11.2).

External appraisers of guidelines can spend many hours trying to re-grade recommendations that have been made, in many cases criticizing the grades that have been awarded because they cannot understand where the link is between the initial evidence and the final recommendation. This process undermines the guideline itself and illustrates two points.

First, that guideline development should be a combination of evidence and clinical experience and involves judgement on the part of the guideline development group.[6,7] Therefore, select the GDG very carefully. People with knowledge and experience need to contribute to the process but the panel needs to be balanced with people holding relatively unbiased opinions.

Second, up to now guideline developers have been simplistic about their approach to the development process and in most cases have not provided stakeholders with information illustrating the judgement that has been involved in the process. This reduces the clarity of the process.

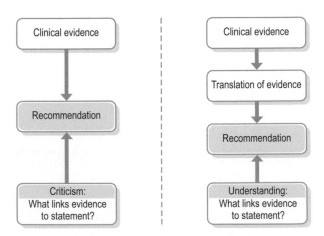

Figure 11.2 Making a recommendation transparent (left side: no explanations of judgement leading to criticisms; right side: explanations of judgement leading to understanding).

Rule 1

Ensure that the guideline development group is explicit about the system employed to translate evidence into a recommendation.

Traditionally only the clinical questions and recommendations have been provided in the final guideline document. More recently a number of institutions (e.g the National Collaborating Centre for Women and Children's Health) have provided clear explanations to demonstrate the link between the evidence and the recommendations (Example Box 11.3).

Rule 2

Ensure that stakeholders have access to the discussions and information forming the basis of the judgements that have been made to translate the evidence into a recommendation if they ask for it – i.e. keep a record of the whole process.

Making recommendations which make sense

It is important that there is no ambiguity about what the recommendation is recommending!

Tips

- Keep recommendations short
- Each recommendation should stand alone
- A recommendation should recommend an action, not be a statement of fact
- The recommendations should follow in the sequence of clinical management
- The sequence of clinical management should be continuous, i.e. no gaps which need to be filled in by guideline users
- If gaps exist due to a lack of research evidence, consider cementing the gaps with formal consensus statements (see Chapters 8 and 9)

113

Example Box 11.3 Illustration of a clear explanation of evidence translation NICE guideline: Feverish illness in children[8]

Clinical question:
What are the clinical symptoms and signs of meningitis in children aged less than 5 with a fever?

Evidence summary:
We found two evidence level 2+ prospective population studies and one evidence level 2− population study to determine the symptoms and signs of bacterial meningitis. Neck stiffness and a decreased conscious level are the best predictors of bacterial meningitis. However, neck stiffness is often absent in infants under 12 months. Infants under 12 months of age have a bulging fontanelle in 55% of bacterial meningitis cases.

Translation:
The GDG considered neck stiffness, a bulging fontanelle and a decreased conscious level as being serious clinical features. The GDG also felt it was important to highlight to healthcare professionals that classic features of meningitis are often absent in infants.

Continued

> **Example Box 11.3** *Continued*
>
> **Recommendation:**
> Meningitis should be considered in a child with fever and any of the following features:
> * neck stiffness;
> * bulging fontanelle;
> * decreased conscious level.
>
> Healthcare professionals should be aware that classical signs of meningitis (neck stiffness, bulging fontanelle, high-pitched cry) are often absent in infants with bacterial meningitis.

Grading recommendations

Over the years there has been an increase in the number of grading systems available. This can cause a great deal of confusion as the same recommendation may be given one grade using one system and another grade using a different system. The individual systems are further described in Chapter 7.

Pros of grading recommendations

As mentioned above, people have traditionally been under the impression that the literature can be appraised and then translated directly into a 'grade' of recommendation reflecting the strength of evidence it was based on. For example, if the literature review appraised a good randomized controlled trial which was rated as level 1 it would become a grade A recommendation (see Table 11.1). By using this grading method the guideline users would know how much confidence to have in the recommendation without needing to know about the evidence underpinning it all.[5]

Cons of grading recommendations

Over time it has become clear through implementation studies and audit that only grade A recommendations are being implemented by local Trusts/services, despite the fact that the consensus recommendations may actually have more impact on practice.

Table 11.1	Relationship between level of evidence and grade of recommendation used by SIGN and NICE[1]

Grade	Type of recommendation
A	Requires at least one meta-analysis, systematic review or RCT rated as 1++, and directly applicable to the target population, and demonstrating overall consistency of results
B	Requires a body of evidence including studies rated as 2++, directly applicable to the target population, and demonstrating overall consistency of results; or extrapolated evidence from studies rated as 1++ or 1+
C	Requires a body of evidence including studies rated as 2+, directly applicable to the target population, and demonstrating overall consistency of results; or extrapolated evidence from studies rated as 2++
D	Evidence level 3 or 4; or extrapolated evidence from studies rated as 2+

With the number of different grading systems developed the guideline user can be confused as to what exactly a grade B or C recommendation means.

Methodologists from NICE and other institutions have come to realize that alternative systems, such as not grading the recommendations at all, may need to be used. By stating the level of evidence and explaining the judgement (or translation) which has been added to the recommendation, the statement should need no grade. Each recommendation then stands as strong as the next.

Grading the next generation of guidelines

One grading system that is increasingly being adopted is the GRADE system.[9] We will briefly describe the process used in the GRADE system.

Step 1

Take the quality of evidence into consideration. The quality of a study can be affected by issues mentioned below.

- Study design – e.g. observational or randomized
- Study quality – i.e. methodological quality
- Consistency – i.e. can the data apply to different subgroups?
- Directness – i.e. do the data apply to the population of interest?

Having taken the above into consideration a study that initially is given a higher grade, for example because it is a randomized controlled trial, may move down a level and a study that is at a lower level may move up.

A simple summary of the evidence is outlined below in Table 11.2.

Step 2

Decide whether the recommendation would be more beneficial or harmful. During this step it is important for the guideline panel not only to consider their own views but to take into account the views of the patients whom their recommendations will affect. It is for this reason that it is vital that the GDG must include patient representation. Cost considerations should ideally be made after this step so that the clinical opinion is safeguarded.

- *Net benefits* – the intervention clearly does more good than harm
- *Trade-offs* – there are important trade-offs between the benefits and harms

Table 11.2	Summary	
	High	Further research is very unlikely to change our confidence in the estimate of effect
	Moderate	Further research is likely to have an important impact on our confidence in the estimate of effect and may change the estimate
	Low	Further research is very likely to have an important impact on our confidence in the estimate of effect and may change the estimate
	Very low	An estimate of effect is very uncertain

- *Uncertain trade-offs* – it is not clear whether the intervention does more good than harm
- *No net benefits* – the intervention clearly does not do more good than harm

The GRADE method, rather than grading the recommendation, provides a very simple way of categorizing recommendations.

- 'Do it' or 'don't do it'
- 'Probably do it' or 'probably don't do it'
- 'No recommendation can be made because there is no clear agreement'.

In all situations a guideline user should take the patient's views into consideration, but one would have more confidence in suggesting an intervention based on a 'do it' recommendation. More negotiation with the patient for a 'probably do it' recommendation would be required.

Summary

- Collect all the evidence, consensus, health data and patient views together.
- Document the judgement used by the GDG.
- Ensure there is no ambiguity in the recommendation.
- Decide how best to communicate the strength of the recommendation to the guideline users.

116

References

1. Scottish Intercollegiate Guidelines Network. SIGN guidelines: an introduction to SIGN methodology for the development of evidence-based clinical guidelines. 1999. Edinburgh. www.sign.ac.uk
2. National Health and Medical Research Council. A guide to the development, implementation and evaluation of clinical practice guidelines. 1998. Canberra: Australian Government Publishing Service.
3. Royal College of Paediatrics and Child Health. Standards for development of clinical guidelines in paediatrics and child health (3rd edn). 2006. RCPCH. www.rcpch.ac.uk
4. Department of Health. Clinical guidelines: Using clinical practice guidelines to improve patient care within the NHS. Leeds: Department of Health; 1996.
5. National Institute of Health and Clinical Excellence. Guideline development methods: information for national collaborating centres and guideline developers. 2004. NICE. www.nice.nhs.uk
6. Sackett D et al. Evidence-based medicine: how to practice and teach EBM. London: Churchill Livingstone; 2000.
7. Margolis C, Cretin S. Implementing clinical practice guidelines. Chicago: American Hospital Association Press; 1999.
8. NICE clinical guideline. Feverish illness in children: assessment and initial management in children up to 5 years. 2007. NICE. www.nice.nhs.uk
9. The Grading of Recommendations Assessment, Development and Evaluation (GRADE) Working Group. Grading quality of evidence and strength of recommendations. BMJ 2004; 328:1490–1493.

Chapter 12

The audit package

Roddy MacFaul

Aims

- To briefly revise the audit cycle
- To describe the inclusion of audit as part of the guideline package
- To describe the use of audit as an implementation tool

Why build audit into a guideline?

Unless you are an accountant, the word 'audit' usually instils a sense of dread or boredom into many of us. This is partly because of the negative, sometimes tedious, aspects of data collection. Perhaps it is also that many small audits are started and never completed or do not lead to recognizable change. However, at the same time as feeling negative about audit, we recognize that clinical audit has an integral and major role in driving improvements in practice. The Healthcare Commission considers 'the purpose of audit is to improve patient outcome by improving professional practice and general quality of services delivered'.[1] The GMC advises all doctors that 'they must take part in regular and systematic medical and clinical audit, recording data honestly'.[2] Similar statements come from the Nursing and Midwifery Council and other healthcare professions' bodies.

Guideline developers also have a key role to play in improving health care. The production and implementation of an evidence-based guideline aims to improve patient outcome by improving practice and the quality of services delivered. The process of auditing a guideline will highlight not only areas where improvement has occurred but also the areas where further practice development is required. Audit of the implemented guideline has to be encouraged.

Encouraging audit, however, is not a passive process. A guideline development group (GDG) needs to break down the audit barriers which local guideline implementers (see Chapter 14) may encounter or perceive. One successful way of encouraging audit is for the GDG to set up an audit package linked to the

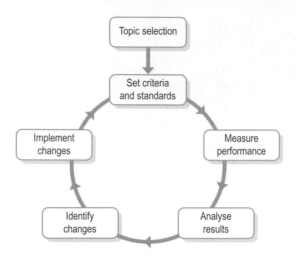

Figure 12.1 Steps in the audit cycle.

guideline documentation. By recommending explicit audit criteria for the guideline and suggesting, or even designing, audit tools for data collection, the local guideline implementers will be able to use this package from the start rather than having to design their own. Half of the barriers to auditing the guideline locally will already be knocked down!

Another advantage of building audit into the guideline is realized when the guideline is being implemented across multiple healthcare providers. Having a standard set of audit criteria allows the meaningful comparison of performance across the different settings. Improvements in standards of care can be encouraged throughout the healthcare community by highlighting role models who perform well and applying their guideline implementation strategy more widely (see Chapter 14).

To add further emphasis to the importance of audit, NICE and SIGN have agreed that audit criteria form an essential component of guideline development. When the guideline is externally appraised before being published it will be assessed on whether audit criteria have been included (see Appendix 1: The AGREE Instrument 'Applicability: The guideline presents key review criteria for monitoring and/or audit purposes'[3]).

The audit cycle

There are several key steps in the audit cycle (Figure 12.1).

Topic selection

The reasons for selecting an audit topic are very similar to those for developing a guideline (see Chapter 4: Getting started). Below are some of the questions you asked before you chose to develop a guideline in this field and now need to audit:

■ Is the topic an important public health problem in terms of numbers, cost or clinical risk?

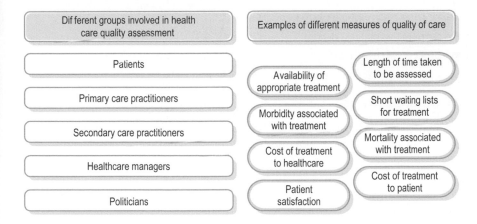

Figure 12.2 Healthcare measures of quality will be prioritized differently by perspectives of what is important to individual groups.

- Is there evidence that the current quality of health care should be improved (e.g. previous audit results, new research findings, risk assessment data)?
- Is there good research evidence available about the most clinically effective and cost-effective management of patients?
- Are there measurable clinical outcomes which can be used to monitor performance?
- Is there enthusiasm to change practice for the better in this area?

The effort required to complete the audit cycle can be considerable. Therefore it is better to prioritize a few key areas for regular, accurate audit than to perform a lot of small, one-off audits which rarely drive change.[4]

Setting criteria and standards

Audit aims to improve the quality of care. 'Quality of care', however, is a difficult beast to pin down. The most important measures of quality of care will be defined differently by different groups at different times (Figure 12.2). Therefore, quality of care cannot easily be measured by a single criterion alone.

Selecting the measure of quality of care is therefore fundamental to the audit process.

Audit criteria

Criteria are 'definable and measurable items of health care which describe quality and which can be used to measure it'.[5] Criteria[6] should:

- be explicit rather than implicit;
- relate to important aspects of care;
- be measurable;
- be evidence-based including the use of consensus methods where necessary;
- have some pre-assessment of likely achievement.

Audit criteria can often be categorized into:

■ structure (what you need);

■ process (what you do);

■ outcome (what you expect).

Structure criteria

Structure criteria refer to the infrastructure of the service, i.e. the premises and equipment, staff and training, IT systems. Because one purpose of audit is to identify any impediments to delivery of high-quality care, some structure criteria should be included. They are likely to show differences in the clinical environment in which different teams are working when applying the guideline. Thus structure audit points may both explain the performance rating of another criterion or outcome and show where change is needed (Example Box 12.1). Structure items include:

■ ways in which patients access care;

■ quality of records, staff or equipment;

■ treatment resources.

Example Box 12.1	Structure criteria for audit NICE guideline: Self-harm[7]
Recommendation	Trusts provide adequate training for healthcare staff who have contact with people who self-harm.
Evidence	Level 4 – based on focus groups, qualitative research and expert opinion.
Audit criteria	Training includes: • the problems faced by people who self-harm when they have contact with services • an exploration of some of the meanings and motives for self-harm • capacity and consent in relation to self-harm • assessment of people who self-harm • early management, including the use of activated charcoal • the content of the NICE guideline
Implementation of guideline	After the publication of the guideline, the Department of Health issued an implementation tool and a benchmarking scheme to emergency departments.[8] This contained specific recommendations on training and data were collated centrally. Role models have been highlighted in this benchmarking scheme so that staff are empowered to improve their training if necessary.
Comment	• This audit criterion relates to quality of staff in a system, measured by their training levels. The assumption is made that if staff have been trained in self-harm issues they will use them when they encounter a service user who has self-harmed. The quality of care markers for patients who have self-harmed includes being treated with respect and care. Improving this marker may be best achieved by staff training. Auditing the availability of training for staff (or the percentage of staff who have been trained) is an incentive to initiate training programmes and improve the quality of care for this patient group. Training is measurable and achievable within the NHS, so can be a useful audit criterion.

Process criteria

Process criteria can provide direct measures of quality of care and can also act in some cases as proxy measures of outcome. Criteria used include:

- time taken to access care;
- appropriate clinical assessment, and investigations performed to reach the diagnosis;
- treatments given (or inappropriate ones avoided).

All of these should be supported by good communication and records, which can also be subject to audit as a proxy for outcome or simply 'good care'.

Where research evidence confirms that clinical care processes have an influence on outcome, measurement of the process of care can provide a direct proxy for outcome and thus reduce the need for outcome measures. They have the appeal that they are based on what the clinical team is doing and, importantly, they are usually within the team's control to influence. Thus feedback on this type of criterion becomes more meaningful (Example Box 12.2).

Process measures are easier to measure and to identify. There are also more of them to choose from. They can provide early feedback during the audit cycle. However, their choice should be related to important aspects of care and not be selected simply

Example Box 12.2	Process criteria for audit *NICE guideline: Chronic obstructive pulmonary disease (COPD)*[9]
Recommendation	All health professionals managing COPD should have access to spirometry and be competent in the interpretation of the results.
Evidence	1. Spirometry results form part of the definition of COPD (level 4) 2. Smoking cessation improves outcome in patients with COPD (level 1a) 3. Smoking cessation is increased by patients knowing their spirometry results (level 1b)
Audit criterion	Percentage of patients with COPD who have had spirometry performed.
Implementation of guideline	When the guideline was published the new contract for UK GPs meant that performing spirometry became a key target with financial rewards.[10] The majority of UK GP practices now have access to spirometry.
Comment	• This audit criterion relates to appropriate assessment of patients, measured by whether they have or have not had spirometry performed. The assumptions are that if spirometry has been performed then the treating practitioner has access to a spirometer (part of the structure of the service) and the feedback to the patient may encourage smoking cessation (an important outcome).
	This process criterion is easier to measure for individuals than centrally determining the availability of spirometry across a region (structure criteria). It is also a proxy measure of outcome. A pure outcome criterion could be measured e.g. 'Percentage of patients who stop smoking within 3 months of spirometry'. This criterion would be less easy to measure and would be less under the direct control of those delivering quality health care. Performing a test is a measurable process criterion and can be implemented by shop-floor practitioners if the structure of the service is in place to do so.

because they are more easily counted or recorded. Their inclusion should be justified and comprehensible to users of the guideline.

Outcome criteria

The aim of improving the quality of care is to improve the outcome of patients affected by various diseases. Measuring outcome criteria can be difficult – though not impossible. From the available NICE guidelines, there are only a couple with outcome criteria suggested as topics for audit (Example Box 12.3).

Example Box 12.3 Outcome criteria for audit
NICE guideline: Caesarean section[11]

Recommendation	No specific recommendation, but it is generally noted that caesarean section rates vary dramatically across different healthcare settings (from 4% to 59% of pregnant women had a caesarean before labour in England and Wales).
Evidence	A national audit of caesarean rates[12] compared local rates of caesarean to the national average. Grade 1++ evidence of ways to improve the number of normal vaginal births and therefore reduce maternal and fetal morbidity/mortality.
Audit criteria	Hospitals should measure the overall caesarean rates as well as the percentage of caesarean sections performed for the four major determinants (presumed fetal compromise, failure to progess in labour, breech presentation, multiple pregnancy) and 'maternal request'.
Implementation of guideline	Evidence-based guidance was provided nationally on management of labour including the need to perform a caesarean. Collecting data on caesarean rates was already part of a national audit[12] which most maternity units subscribed to.
Comment	• This audit criterion simply measures the outcome of delivery. There is an assumption that the rate of caesarean section is under the control of the staff in maternity units. By measuring the percentage of caesareans performed, feedback is given to staff on how well they have implemented the guideline's other recommendations. • The evidence that outcome of women post caesarean is worse compared to a normal vaginal delivery is clear. Therefore, caesareans should only be performed when there is an identifiable indication. Auditing the percentage of women who have a caesarean without an identifiable indication should encourage staff to investigate why caesareans are being performed in these cases. This is a useful measure of guideline implementation and validation. If the caesarean rate falls in a unit where the recommendations have been applied then the staff will continue to implement the guideline – positive feedback. Role models for guideline implementation can be identified and highlighted for other units to follow. This outcome measure is also readily measurable. Data are already routinely collected on mode of delivery of pregnant women and the indication is also routinely documented. This outcome can also be affected by shop-floor practitioners who make the decision to intervene or not.

Audit aims to rapidly feed back ways to improve health care to the staff providing that care. Completion of the audit cycle in a reasonable time period is especially important so that feedback to clinical staff can occur indicating the need for change. Rare outcomes will be difficult to use as audit criteria, as once enough data have been established, practice or even the staff may have changed. This will reduce the relevance of the results to those caring for the current patient population. For example, selecting the audit criterion of death as an outcome measure of quality of care in treating community acquired pneumonia in children[13] would be interesting as it is a serious outcome. However, it is so rare in the UK that it would not realistically inform the staff of how to change practice. A better outcome measure would be the outcome of developing a complication such as an empyema or the length of hospital stay.

Long-term outcomes are similarly difficult to incorporate into an audit. However, if evidence is available linking short-term outcomes to longer-term outcomes (e.g. cardiac exercise testing at 6 weeks post myocardial infarction is related to cardiac deaths at 1 year[14]) then these should be considered for audit.

Outcomes are dependent on many factors. These may not always be influenced by the process of care – however high quality – because of variation in severity of the initial illness, presence of co-morbidities or social factors outside the influence of the providing clinical service. Choosing an outcome criterion in a guideline audit will require significant resources in 'drilling down' through the data to understand the root cause of any poor outcomes. As well as patient population variation, it may reflect the deficiencies in the structure of the service, variation in practice or variation in practitioner performance. If the outcome criterion is outside the control of the healthcare workers (e.g. smoking cessation rates in COPD patients offered spirometry) then it will not necessarily help to improve the quality of care – it will just be information.

Standards

Standards (benchmarks or targets) are levels of care to be achieved for any particular audit criterion. They are the numerical value of performance, e.g. the criterion for audit is measuring the number of patients with COPD who have spirometry recorded; the standard for quality of care is that 80% of COPD patients have spirometry recorded. The criterion is fixed but the standard can be variable (e.g. in different healthcare settings, or in different audit cycles).

The numerical standard can be set by:

- evidence;
- knowledge of current performance;
- consensus.

Ideally standards should be set by research findings, e.g. the target percentage of women who should have their babies delivered by caesarean section could be set by the incidence of the various indications for caesareans including presumed fetal compromise, failure to progress in labour, breech presentation and multiple pregnancy. But defining standards fully justified by evidence poses a particular challenge. Some may be easier than others depending on the evidence available (Example Box 12.4).

Example Box 12.4 Setting standards using evidence
Newborn blood spot screening in the UK[15]

Recommendation	Babies with congenital hypothyroidism (CHT) or phenylketonuria (PKU) should start treatment for these conditions before 21 days of life.
Evidence	High-quality cohort data on the neurological outcome of children with these conditions depending on the time of commencing treatment – level 2++ [16–18]
Audit criteria	1. Sample collection – percentage of blood spot samples obtained between days 5 and 8
	2. Sample dispatch – percentage of blood spot samples reaching labs within 4 working days of sample being taken
	3. Untested babies – percentage of babies identified as not tested or declined the test by day 19
	4. Processing of positive screening tests – percentage of positive screening tests being processed within 4 working days of laboratory receiving sample
Standards	1. Sample collection
	○ Core standard: 95% of first samples taken between 5 and 8 days (ideally day 5)
	○ Developmental standard: 100% of first samples taken between 5 and 8 days (ideally day 5)
	2. Sample dispatch
	○ Core standard: 100% of samples received by laboratory within 4 working days of sample being taken
	○ Developmental standard: 100% of samples received by laboratory within 2 working days of sample being taken
	3. Untested babies
	○ Core standard: 100% of untested babies (including declined) identified by day 19
	○ Developmental standard: 100% of untested babies (including declined) identified by day 14
	4. Processing of positive screening tests
	○ Core standard: 100% of positive screening results available and clinical referral made within 4 working days of sample receipt
	○ Developmental standard: 100% of positive screening results available and clinical referral made within 3 working days of sample receipt

If there are no data either from research or from previous audit work, consensus may be used to determine a standard. However, it's all too easy to recommend 100% targets, which in reality will rarely be met – unless the incentives are substantial (i.e. financial). Pie-in-the-sky standards could lead to a sense of failure and despondency in the clinical teams performing the audit.

The Department of Health has suggested recently that placing a value on a standard should be done at two levels:[19]

- a core standard – setting out the minimum level of service expected by patients;
- a developmental standard – the goal to be achieved through improvements in service.

It may also be reasonable not to place a value on a standard initially. If there is no information to guide a standard, why guess at one? Once audit data are available then by averaging the results from different healthcare providers a core standard

Methods of data collection		
Retrospectively	vs	Prospectively
Routine data collection methods	vs	Specifically designed data collection sheets
Data collected by one investigator	vs	Multiple staff members collecting data

Examples of national audits using specifically designed audit collection sheets		
Organization	**Information collected**	**Infrastructure**
PICANet(Paediatric Intensive Care Audit Network)	Patient details and admission details for children on PICUs	Results collated centrally; IT program to make data entry simple
NHS Information Authority – Head and neck cancer care	Patient demographics and hospital care provided	Results collated centrally; pilot programme to assess audit tools
National Asthma Campaign	Patient details and documented hospital care/follow-up	Results collated centrally; electronic data entry and analysis

could be assigned for the next audit cycle. The developmental standard in the next audit cycle could be that achieved by the best performing centre in the first audit.

125

Measuring performance

Data collection should be an easy process! We all know though that this is probably the most challenging area of audit.

Data can be collected in a number of ways (Table 12.1).

Using retrospective methods will lead to headaches trying to identify cases. Diagnostic codes are frequently inadequate to capture the patients you are interested in. Trying to obtain the notes will be time consuming. If cases can be retrospectively identified and the notes found, trying to decipher the information required for the audit from the documentation made at the time will not always be straightforward.

Similarly, routinely kept patient data will rarely be sufficient for completing an audit. Specifically designed data collection sheets are used for major national audits, many of which are so well established that they have become 'routine' to those filling them in (Table 12.2).

When designing a data collection sheet it is vital to:

■ keep it short;

■ keep it simple;

■ pilot it;

■ adapt it;

■ keep it short again.

Keep it short

As audit means extra work in terms of data collection, the data collection sheet has to be straightforward enough for anybody to fill in, short enough that it will be completed and comprehensive enough that it will provide adequate information for the audit criteria. It can be all too tempting to suggest adding another box for data entry because 'it would be interesting to know'. Be focused on the remit of the audit.

Keep it simple

Try to use objective measures for data entry, e.g. respiratory rate on admission, rather than subjective measures, e.g. patient breathless yes/no. If subjective assessments have to be included in audit then ideally samples of cases should be subjected to double reporting and the inter-observer reliability checked with methods such as the kappa statistic.

Pilot

Pilot it – maybe several times – and analyse the results on a small scale before suggesting other units use this tool. Where clinical data are being obtained for audit purposes it is vital that single questions which have no ambiguity are used for data extraction. PICANet took several months to perfect their data collection forms. One piece of information collected was the number of days children on PICUs were intubated for.[20] Several centres found the wording of a draft form confusing – did being intubated from 11.45 p.m. on Tuesday to 3.30 a.m. on Wednesday mean the child was intubated for zero days (not a full 24 hours), 1 day, or 2 days (as the patient was intubated on Tuesday and Wednesday)? These issues need to be ironed out as soon as they are highlighted.

Adapt

By analysing the results of a few patients in a pilot audit, it should be possible to determine whether you have the right data to answer the original audit criteria. If you need a different bit of information to answer the question then change and re-pilot the form.

Information technology may speed up the process of audit. If the data entry forms are electronic or readable by computer then data extraction will be faster and so feedback of the analysed results will be rapid. A rapid turnaround from data collection to feedback will probably help motivate practitioners to complete the audit cycle!

How many patients or how long should data be collected for? This is an arbitrary figure but is related to the expected frequency of encountering a patient who fits the guideline – and therefore audit – criteria and to the number needed to provide a meaningful and valid answer in the analysis. It will be practically limited by practitioner fatigue – data will be collected enthusiastically for a finite period unless sufficient carrots or sticks are present.

When developing the audit package to complement the guideline, it is important to state any special circumstances, that will exclude patients from an audit criterion. This will reduce the risk that patient mix is the cause for variation in performance by different healthcare providers.

Care pathways (see Appendix 2) can provide a neat solution to both data collection for audit and guideline implementation (see Chapter 14). If a care pathway is designed around the guideline and this forms part of the clinical documentation, then hopefully not only will practitioners be reminded to implement key guideline recommendations as they manage a patient, but they will also be filling in the data for the various audit criteria as part of the patient documentation. The care pathway can simply be photocopied at the end of the patient episode – one copy to the notes and one to audit.

Analyse results

The guideline development group needs to decide whether they are going to analyse the data centrally or encourage local guideline implementers to analyse their own results. Central analysis has the advantage that national performance targets can be established and an atmosphere of healthy competition among healthcare providers drives improvements. However, there may be significant costs in setting up the infrastructure for central analysis (Example Box 12.5).

If there is no feedback of audit results to the guideline development group, then implementation strategies will be slower to evolve and the guideline will remain a static document, rather than a dynamic process. A guideline should improve with time as new evidence of best practice is incorporated. This includes the evidence from audit on how best to implement the guideline in the workplace.

Identify changes

Two elements need to be identified:

- changes in the service to improve performance;
- changes to the guideline.

Service changes

On the whole, people respond less well to being told what to do than being encouraged to do something. Therefore identifying changes in practice should really be left to the local guideline implementers. They have the knowledge of their service structure and processes, e.g. limited out-of-hours access to CT affecting the implementation of the NICE head injury guideline.[21] The GDG can highlight model healthcare providers, thereby allowing comparisons between service providers. Those who are unsure where to make changes may be able to contrast their practices with others who have better patient outcomes.

Guideline changes

If all the healthcare providers who participated in the guideline implementation and audit process perform poorly on the same audit criteria, it may be that the problem lies with the guideline. Perhaps the recommendation is not understood, perhaps it is not being implemented because it is not evidence-based, perhaps there is new evidence yet to be incorporated into the guideline, perhaps the audit criteria are not good markers of healthcare quality or perhaps the whole country has poor healthcare in this area. The GDG should look back at the guideline and review the recommendations.

Example Box 12.5 Central analysis of an audit of a national guideline

Organization	The National Asthma Campaign UK (NACUK)[22]
Guideline	British guidelines for the management of asthma[23]
Audit criteria (included)	Acute hospital admissions: • percentage of patients discharged with a personalized asthma management plan documented in notes • percentage of patients discharged with an assessment of inhaler technique documented in notes
Data collection	Prospective data collection locally at multiple sites (identified through Royal Colleges specialists register) over 1 month in 2001 Piloted data collection sheet = two sides A4
Data analysis	Microsoft Access program used to analyze data electronically Data summarized locally then sent to central register in Glasgow
Report	Local performance summarized and compared to national average Practice in top performing units highlighted to encourage change and improvement
Re-audit	To be announced when further funding
Difficulties overcome	Ethical approval not required as individual patient data collected locally and not identifiable centrally; individual performance of hospitals not published (publication of an audit requires ethical approval)

Implement changes

If the audit is centrally analysed and implemented then before re-auditing enough time has to be given to the local units to implement any changes (see Chapter 14).

Set criteria and standards again

By this stage (completing the audit cycle) new evidence may have become available and results of audit may also indicate a need for changes in the guideline. Knowing that the guideline will evolve with time means that criteria selected for re-audit should include those which are more likely to remain stable over the period of an audit cycle. If the goalposts keep moving because the recommendations keep changing, then improvements over time in clinical care will be difficult to detect. Comparative audit is more meaningful if the same criterion is used again and again.

Standards can be reset and reassessed with the knowledge of performance in the first audit.

Tips

Tasks for a GDG to set up an audit package:

1. Select criteria and set standards – use meaningful process criteria that are measurable
2. Design a care pathway for the guideline, so structured record will make data collection automatic

   or

   Design and pilot data collection sheets

> 3. Consider central analysis of data
>   - IT services will be available (e.g. Microsoft Access programs) to make this straightforward
>   - Ensure that feedback is rapid
> 4. Identify audit leads locally
>   - Royal College lists
>   - Clinical effectiveness networks
>   - Specialist associations
> 5. Ensure that a system is set up for guideline review with knowledge of audit results

Using audit as an implementation tool

Guideline implementation is not an easy task (see Chapter 14). It requires a number of elements including:

- advertising the existence of the guideline;
- teaching the use of the guideline;
- identifying key local opinion leaders to help encourage the use of the guideline on the shop floor;
- positive feedback for using the guideline;
- reminders to keep using the guideline;
- demonstration that the guideline improves practice.

Setting up an audit scheme for the guideline may help with many of the implementation requirements above and may need fewer resources than you might think (see Tips box above).

Advertising the guideline

You will already have spent considerable effort on telling people about the guideline. Asking people to audit the guideline will remind them that it exists and encourage them to use it before they start collecting data (no-one wants to be audited unfavourably).

Teaching guideline use

During the audit process, the criteria chosen will become very familiar to those filling in the data collection sheets. Staff often talk about the audits which are going on in their department and will therefore have a raised awareness of the existence of the guideline and how to use it.

Identifying a local opinion leader

Most healthcare departments have a lead for audit. If you have not identified a clinical lead for implementing the guideline, then using the audit lead is another avenue. If they are incentivized to audit the guideline (e.g. by providing the audit package to go with the guideline; by coordinating results centrally for comparison of their performance against others), then they will also be keen to implement the guideline.

Positive feedback

Audit is one of the best ways of feeding back performance to staff. Positive feedback will encourage continued use of the guideline's recommendations. Staff are not necessarily rewarded only if they are performing at the highest level. The reward for staff is often simply knowing how they are performing.

Reminders

Re-audit will remind members of staff that there are sound recommendations for practice and to continue using them.

Demonstrating that guideline use improves practice

Even if the guideline is rigorously constructed and evidence-based throughout, some professionals will not want to implement the guideline until they know it has an impact. Audit can demonstrate that implementing a guideline will improve quality of care (Example Box 12.6). An audit of practice before a guideline is available followed by a period of implementation then re-auditing the same criteria will provide powerful evidence of the value of guideline implementation.

Example Box 12.6	Audit as an implementation tool – demonstration of changes in practice by implementing a guideline	
Guideline	Diarrhoea and vomiting – an evidence-based guideline for children presenting with diarrhoea with or without vomiting[24]	
Recommendation	Oral rehydration should be the standard treatment for children with mild to moderate dehydration secondary to gastroenteritis – Evidence level 1++	
Audit criteria	Percentage of children in each category of dehydration (mild/moderate/severe) who have a cannula sited with or without commencement of IV rehydration	
Standard	Only children with severe dehydration or failed oral/NG rehydration should have a cannula sited and IV rehydration started	
Data	Pre-implementation	Post-implementation
Number seen	292	239
No. with severe dehydration	0	1
% admitted	27%	34%
% started IV rehydration	15%	2%
Comment	After the implementation of the guideline there was a dramatic reduction in the use of IV rehydration, thereby reducing risk and harm to the patients and cost to the healthcare service	

Summary

- Audit criteria and data collection tools should be developed alongside the guideline recommendations.
- Developing a care pathway would help both implementation and audit.
- Central analysis of data allows for quality of care comparisons across different healthcare providers.
- The guideline should be reviewed in the light of audit results.

References

1. Commission for Healthcare Audit and Inspection. What is clinical audit? London: Commission for Healthcare Audit and Inspection, The Stationery Office; 2004. www.healthcarecommission.org.uk
2. General Medical Council. Good medical practice. London: General Medical Council; 2001. www.gmc-uk.org
3. Appraisal of Guidelines for Research and Evaluation (AGREE) Instrument. The AGREE Collaboration. 2001. www.agreecollaboration.org.
4. John C, Mathew D, Gnanalingham M. An audit of paediatric audits. Arch Dis Child 2004; 89:1130.
5. Irvine D, Irvine S (eds) Making sense of audit. Oxford: Radcliffe Medical Press; 1991.
6. National Institute for Clinical Excellence. Principles for best practice in clinical audit. London: National Institute for Clinical Excellence, The Stationery Office; 2002. www.nice.org.uk
7. National Institute for Clinical Excellence. Self-harm: the short-term physical and psychological management and secondary prevention of self-harm in primary and secondary care. NICE Clinical Guideline No. 16. London: National Institute for Clinical Excellence. 2004. www.nice.org.uk
8. Department of Health. Improving the management of patients with mental ill health in emergency care settings. London: Department of Health; 2004. www.dh.gov.uk
9. National Institute for Clinical Excellence. Chronic obstructive pulmonary disease – Management of chronic obstructive pulmonary disease in adults in primary and secondary care. NICE Clinical Guideline No. 12. London: National Institute for Clinical Excellence; 2004. www.nice.org.uk
10. Department of Health. Primary care contracting. Quality and outcomes framework – guidance updated August 2004. London: Department of Health; 2004. www.dh.gov.uk
11. National Institute for Clinical Excellence. Caesarean section. NICE Clinical Guideline No. 13. London: National Institute for Clinical Excellence; 2004. www.nice.org.uk
12. Thomas J, Paranjothy S, Royal College of Obstetricians and Gynaecologists Clinical Effectiveness Support Unit. National Sentinel Caesarean Section Audit Report. London: RCOG Press; 2001.
13. British Thoracic Society Standard of Care Committee. BTS guidelines for the management of community acquired pneumonia in childhood. Thorax 2002; 57:i1-i24.
14. Newby LK et al. Early discharge in the thrombolytic era: an analysis of criteria for uncomplicated infarction from the Global Utilization of Streptokinase and t-PA for Occluded Coronary Arteries (GUSTO) trial. J Am Coll Cardiol 1996; 27(3):625–632.
15. UK Newborn Screening Programme Centre. Policies and standards for newborn blood spot screening. London: Department of Health; 2005. www.newbornscreening-bloodspot.org.uk
16. Medical Research Council. Recommendations on the dietary management of phenylketonuria. Report of the MRC Working Party on Phenylketonuria. Arch Dis Child 1993; 68:426–427.
17. Smith I. Treatment of phenylalanine hydroxylase deficiency. Acta Paediatr Suppl 1994; 407:60–65.
18. Virtanen M et al. Congenital hypothyroidism: age at start of treatment versus outcome. Acta Paediatr Scand 1983; 72:197–201.
19. Department of Health. Standards for better health. London: Department of Health; 2004. www.dh.gov.uk
20. Newsletter May 2003. Paediatric Intensive Care Audit Network 2003. www.picanet.org.uk

21. National Institute for Clinical Excellence. Head injury – triage, assessment, investigation and early management of head injury in infants, children and adults. NICE Clinical Guideline No. 4. London: National Institute for Clinical Excellence; 2003. www.nice.org.uk

22. National Asthma Campaign UK. Asthma audit 2002: an audit of children's asthma in the UK. Asthma J 2002; 8(2 suppl):1–12.

23. SIGN. The British guideline on the management of asthma. Guideline No. 63. Scottish Intercollegiate Guidelines Network. 2004. www.sign.ac.uk

24. Armon K, Stephenson T, MacFaul R et al. An evidence and consensus based guideline for acute diarrhoea management. Arch Dis Child 2001; 85:132–142.

Appraisal

Richard Bowker

Aims

- To suggest appraisal options
- To describe the appraisal tool for guidelines in detail
- To prepare the final guideline for appraisal

133

External appraisal of the fully developed guideline is vital for encouraging implementation of the recommendations. If no independent body has appraised the work, then many practitioners will just turn round and ask why should they use these personal practice recommendations?

Preparing for external appraisal of the guideline takes a little thought. However, if you've been organized during the development process then all the elements should be in place to simply bring together into a guideline document.

Appraisal options

Selecting who to appraise the developed guideline should not be a difficult task. If the guideline is for local use only, then the document will need to be scrutinized by the local guideline committee. Every Trust should have such a committee and its members shouldn't be too difficult to find.

If the guideline has been developed at a national level, then the guideline committee of the appropriate Royal College should be asked to appraise and hopefully endorse the guideline findings. It is always helpful to inform the appraising body at the beginning of the guideline development process that a guideline is being written, so that they can feel a part of it and arrange their appraisal workload appropriately. If the guideline covers more than one specialty, there is every reason to ask more than one College to appraise the document. This may lead to wider dissemination and implementation.

NICE and SIGN produce their own guidelines and do not appraise other people's work. Don't be under the illusion that, by following the rigorous criteria of guideline

Table 13.1

Attributes of high-quality guidelines[1]	
Valid	Correctly interpreting the available evidence so that implementing recommendations leads to improvements in health
Reproducible	With the same evidence, a different guideline development group would produce similar recommendations
Reliable	With the same clinical situation, another healthcare professional would apply the recommendations similarly
Representative	All key disciplines and interests, including patients, have contributed to the guideline's development
Clinically applicable	The target population is similar to the research population, on whose findings the recommendations have been based
Clinically flexible	The guideline identifies where exceptions to the recommendations lie and indicates how patient decisions are to be included
Clearly expressed	The guideline uses precise definitions, unambiguous language and is user-friendly
Well documented	The methodology used is transparent and the evidence is clearly linked to the recommendations
Schedule for review	There is a set date for review and who and how that process will take place

development, the guideline can 'become' a NICE guideline or a SIGN guideline. It just doesn't work like that.

Appraisal tools

There are several appraisal tools which guideline appraisers can use. All the tools aim to assess guidelines objectively on the features described in Table 13.1.

The currently favoured tool is the AGREE Instrument (see Appendix 1). This uses a simple marking form, which ideally two independent reviewers should complete.[2] The categories for marking are:

- scope and purpose;
- stakeholder involvement;
- rigour of development;
- clarity and presentation;
- applicability;
- editorial independence.

For further details on how the AGREE Instrument is used see Appendix 1.

Preparing the guideline document

Appraisal is meant to be an objective process. However, the easier a guideline is to appraise, the more likely the assessor will appraise it in a good frame of mind.

Example Box 13.1 Guideline for the management of decreased conscious level in children[3]
Structure of guideline document

- Acknowledgements
  - Funding
  - Guideline development group
  - Patient involvement
  - Stakeholder groups
  - Delphi panellists
- Index of contents
- Introduction
- Aims
- Scope
- Guideline methodology
  - Participants
  - Clinical questions
  - Evidence search
  - Evidence appraisal
  - Delphi consensus process
  - Economic evaluation
  - Good practice points
  - Recommendation formation
  - Review process
- Guideline recommendations with explanations
- Guideline algorithm
- Implementation strategy
- Audit
- Research points
- Update process
- References
- Appendices
  - Evidence tables
  - Guideline group meetings
  - Delphi consensus results
  - Stakeholder involvement
  - Patient participation

In other words, structure the guideline document in such a way as to highlight the methodology which is important for appraisal.

In Example Box 13.1 (Guideline for the management of decreased conscious level in children), the guideline document is laid out so that the appraiser should be able to find all the information easily.

The document should be transparent in terms of:

- how it was funded;
- who was involved;
- what was the scope of the guideline;
- how the evidence was searched and appraised;
- what evidence was used;
- what judgements went into recommendations;

- what are the audit and research points;
- when and how the guideline is being updated.

Keep the document understandable for the casual reader by using appendices. Search strategies, evidence tables and stakeholder involvement details all need to be present somewhere to make the development process transparent. However, these parts of the document are large and do not make for easy reading – hence the benefit of placing them in an appendix.

Ensure that the evidence is presented in a format which is understandable to the outside reviewer. Keep the evidence tables structured and well referenced (see Chapter 7).

Finally, ensure that the appraiser has the guideline developers' contact details. They may have important queries which if not answered may lead to a less favourable appraisal.

Using the external appraisal

Having undergone external appraisal, it is important to make use of the results.

- *Making changes.* Just like stakeholder contributions, there may be alterations suggested by the appraisers. The GDG will need to give careful consideration to any changes, whether superficial or more serious.

- *Promotion.* Highlight to the end-users that the guideline has been appraised by a responsible professional body. Ask if you can use their crest on the guideline document.

- *Dissemination.* Is there an official publication through which the appraisal can be disseminated? For example, the Royal College of Paediatrics and Child Health publishes all the guidelines it appraises for its members. Other colleges have website versions of guideline appraisals, which can be used to publicize the existence of the guideline.

Summary

- External appraisal is a vital part of the guideline validation process, which will aid implementation.
- Be familiar at the beginning of the development process with the appraisal tool (e.g. AGREE) which the assessors will use.
- Write the guideline document in a way to make appraisal as easy as possible and still be readable by guideline users.

References

1. NHS Centre for Reviews and Dissemination. Implementing clinical practice guidelines: Can guidelines be used to improve clinical practice? Effective Health Care Bulletin, Vol. 1, No. 8. 1994.
2. Appraisal of Guidelines for Research and Evaluation (AGREE) Instrument. The AGREE Collaboration. 2001. www.agreecollaboration.org
3. The Paediatric Accident and Emergency Research Group. Evidence-based guidelines for the management of a child with a decreased conscious level. 2005. www.nottingham. ac.uk/paediatric-guideline

Chapter 14

Dissemination and implementation – or getting the message across

Monica Lakhanpaul

Aims

- To understand the difference between dissemination and implementation
- To describe the different methods employed to disseminate and implement the final guideline
- To understand the long-term input required for implementation of guidelines

Before you publish the final guideline, be under no illusion, the hardest task is yet to come. We are all aware of departmental guidelines that have remained unused on dusty shelves despite the vast amount of effort spent on developing them.

Guidelines which are produced at a national level have to be implemented at the local level.[1] The developers of the guideline do not always bring about their implementation. However, if clinicians on the shop floor fail to use the guideline, then the guideline has failed. Changing the behaviour and practice of healthcare staff is not a passive process. With this realization, organizations such as the Royal Colleges and NICE have turned their attention to active implementation strategies.

Diffusion, dissemination or implementation – what is the difference?

- *Diffusion* is the spreading of information, e.g. by publishing information in a journal. This has not been found to be an effective way of changing clinicians' behaviour but is still an important way of raising awareness of the guideline.[2] The media may also be employed as a tool for diffusing the recommendations. If the stamp of approval has been given by the Royal Colleges (see Chapter 13: Appraisal), then they may have some responsibility for advertising the existence of the guideline.

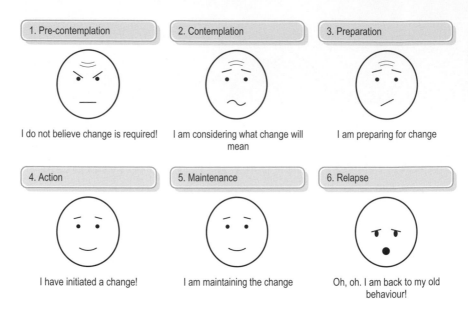

1. Pre-contemplation

I do not believe change is required!

2. Contemplation

I am considering what change will mean

3. Preparation

I am preparing for change

4. Action

I have initiated a change!

5. Maintenance

I am maintaining the change

6. Relapse

Oh, oh. I am back to my old behaviour!

Figure 14.1 The 'transtheoretical model' of behaviour change.[3]

- *Dissemination* is a process used to raise the awareness of the existence of the guideline, its content and the reasons for using it. Compared with diffusion, dissemination involves an element of training. The guideline authors may impart the information by providing individual teaching sessions, small group seminars or presenting at larger conferences. It is unlikely, however, that dissemination of a guideline alone will be sufficient to bring about a change in practice.[2]

- *Implementation* is a more active process and aims to bring about a change in behaviour. A variety of techniques can be tried to encourage health professionals to actually use the recommendations in guidelines, rather than just reading them. Successful guideline implementation strategies result in the adoption of sound research findings in everyday practice.[2]

Understanding people's behaviour

Whether health professionals implement guideline recommendations is closely linked to the way people acquire knowledge, learn and then change their behaviour in accordance with the knowledge they have gained.

A model used in health behavioural sciences has been described to help explain how people change their smoking habits.[3] Individuals pass through a number of stages before they change their behaviour (Figure 14.1), from the ardent smoker who doesn't want to quit, through to the ex-smoker who is tempted to start again in a smoky environment.

This model could be extended to think about how health professionals change their practice (although this has not been validated). Having an idea of which stage an individual is in may help target the most efficient strategy for promoting further change. For example, a practitioner who doesn't believe change is required should be

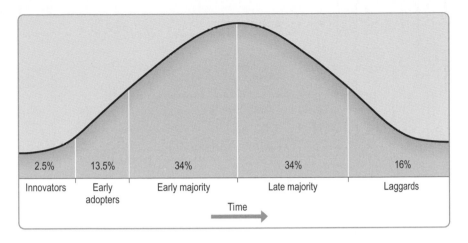

Figure 14.2 The adoption of new ideas at different rates depends on group characteristics.[4]

given information about why there is a problem with current practice and what the advantages are of changing to new ways. Meanwhile, a practitioner who is preparing for change will benefit from information about what needs doing to organize the change in their department and what has worked well elsewhere.

Individuals and institutions are receptive to changes in behaviour at different rates.[1] They may be grouped as *innovators, early adopters, early majority, late majority*, and *laggards* depending on the speed at which change is achieved (Figure 14.2). Don't get disheartened if implementation is not immediate – it may be that you are dealing with a laggard!

Incorporating implementation strategies into guideline development

Facilitating a change in behaviour is a complex process. Individuals will be stimulated to change their behaviour in different ways. Using multi-faceted approaches to target a variety of behaviours is a more successful implementation strategy than an approach concentrating on only one type of intervention alone,[2,5] i.e. hit them from all sides!

Remember, the implementation process begins as soon as the guideline development process begins! A step-by-step approach can be followed to help incorporate implementation strategies into the guideline development process (Figure 14.3). An example of how a national guideline was implemented locally is provided in Example Box 14.1 at the end of this chapter.

1. Highlight current practice

An audit of current practice will highlight differences or deficiencies and suggest areas requiring standardization or improvement. This is usually the initial step to prioritize the development of a specific clinical guideline. This audit information

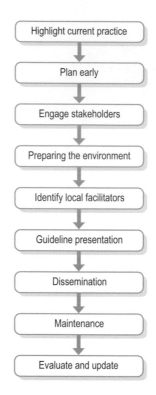

Figure 14.3 Step-by-step approach to successful implementation.

can also be used to encourage a larger group of health professionals that change is required.

Other information sources which can promote change by highlighting current practice include published research findings for novel treatments not currently recommended, patient groups demanding new treatments/services, and media stories around individual cases.

2. Plan implementation strategies early

Think about the strategies for dissemination and implementation at the outset.[2] This requires an investigation into the potential barriers and potential incentives (or driving forces) to using the guideline's recommendations.[6] Some barriers may also be drivers in different circumstances (Table 14.1).

Once the barriers and driving forces to implementation have been identified, develop a plan to overcome or utilize them[6] (see below).

3. Engage stakeholders

Stakeholders include anyone who will use the recommendations or anyone who will need to be involved if the recommendations are used. This may include professionals in primary care, secondary care, or tertiary care. Some of the other groups to

Table 14.1

Barriers and drivers in guideline implementation

Barriers	Factor	Drivers
We don't need to change change	Attitude of local opinion leaders	We would benefit from
We don't believe change is possible	Self-efficacy – confidence in practice one's own abilities	We change to improve all the time
Limited knowledge of guideline recommendations	Publicity and training	Good knowledge of guideline recommendations
Patients won't benefit from change	Evidence base for recommendation	Patients will benefit from change
Our patients don't want to change their care	Patient views	Our patients demand a change to better treatments
Different guidelines say different things	Guideline appraisal	Evidence-based guidelines rigorously developed
Too costly to change	Money	Current practice is expensive. Potential savings in the longer term
We can't change now; we don't have the time to change	Time	Timetable for change in place; change will make our work more efficient
We don't have the skills required for the practice recommended	Education and training	We have the skills in place; we need to obtain new skills for best practice
We don't have the in infrastructure ready	Organizational changes	We have the infrastructure place; our infrastructure is flexible and can accommodate change
We can't see the improvements in service	Positive feedback	The change has notably improved our service
There's nothing in it for us	Reward	We will benefit by changing

consider include administrators, audit and information technologists, and members of the public health team.

Individuals or groups should be identified and involved in the development and implementation process. Identification should be done at the initial scoping stage of the guideline (see Chapter 4: Getting started). Their involvement continues not only until the development process is completed, but through to the guideline's implementation and re-evaluation. Involving stakeholder groups early provides them with a sense of ownership. Ownership will help promote a sense of 'this is our guideline, we will use it' instead of 'this is their guideline, we won't use it as it doesn't apply to us'.

The more disciplines or organizations affected by the guideline, the more important it is to involve them. Multi-professional collaborations are more likely to promote success. Various stakeholders may have conflicting opinions about the content of the guideline. It is pointless to spend vast amounts of time and money on the development process only to find out at the end that one of your key stakeholder groups does not endorse its use! Regularly updating stakeholders on the progress of the guideline and giving them plenty of opportunity to comment on the process should prevent this, and improve the quality of the guideline.

When the guideline is published, the stakeholders represent a large group of individuals who already know about the guideline, and should be willing to promote it to colleagues locally or in their specialty nationally.

Patients/consumers of health services

The UK Department of Health places great emphasis on the identification and inclusion of patient preferences when considering decisions regarding treatment and management of patients.[7] Patients have also been shown to have an effect on the decision-making process of clinicians.[1] It is becoming essential to involve a patient or their representative, when considering strategies for implementation of guidelines.[1]

Just as the stakeholders can have a major effect on the implementation of the guideline, if a guideline does not reflect or consider the needs of the patients, it is unlikely to be successful when put into use. In fact patient groups or charities may actually lobby against its implementation (consider the patient response to the NICE advice on anti-dementia drugs[8]).

As well as including patient representatives during the development stage, producing suitable patient information leaflets to complement the published guideline will help explain the recommendations to patient groups. They in turn may demand the best available treatment, which the guideline recommends, and guideline use by healthcare practitioners.

4. Preparing the environment

Communication and education is the key to success. Local departments need to be informed of the potential introduction of the guideline to allow them time to consider what change will mean. Health professionals do not like to be surprised by introducing change into their already busy and stressful jobs, especially if it going to have a direct effect on the way they manage their patients. The guideline developer responsible for leading the change should be sensitive to these issues.

It is helpful to break the ice by arranging education workshops prior to the implementation of the guideline to familiarize people with the recommendations embedded within the document. Local resources necessary for implementation of guidelines can be identified and potential barriers may be tackled. This is also a good time to identify local facilitators.

5. Identify a local facilitator

Enlisting the help of individuals at a local level and giving them the responsibility of implementing the recommendations locally is essential to the success of the programme. These facilitators should ideally be opinion leaders in their local hospital/practice area, so they can lead change taking their colleagues with them ('I'll do that because she's doing that and I respect her ideas'). Often the lead clinician or practitioner with a responsibility for guidelines can be identified and sweet-talked into helping. The earlier in the process they are identified, the more likely they are to come on board.

These are busy practitioners, so they mustn't be overloaded with too much responsibility or they may become a barrier to change rather than a driver of it. Ensure that they are clear about the key recommendations that need to be implemented, provide them with any material they may need to educate/support the staff involved in the change and listen to feedback from them about how the implementation process is going. Identification of barriers by them may help you to adapt your plans for other centres. Supporting them through the process by showing an interest in how they are doing will also help them to continue making the changes.

6. Presenting the guideline

- *Quality.* Clinical guidelines are more likely to be used if they are evidence-based, simple, flexible, rigorously produced and perceived to improve quality of care.[9] It is important that the quality of the guideline is explicit so that users can trust the recommendations. External appraisal of a guideline (using the AGREE Instrument) will help demonstrate the quality of the guideline development process. If that appraisal has been completed by a well recognized body (e.g. a Royal College or a national special interest group) then that should add further to the quality assurance of the guideline (see Chapter 13: Appraisal).

- *Presentation.* Guidelines need to be easily accessible and presented with clarity. Busy people are unlikely to read something that is very long or complicated. The actual format in which the guideline is presented is therefore extremely important if people are even going to pick it up and read it, never mind use it. Guidelines can be presented in a number of different ways. Assess the format most suitable to the working environment and to the health professionals using them. The earlier this is thought about the fewer draft formats will need to be designed, refined and then finally consigned to the bin!

Examples of styles

- A 'key recommendations' document (kept in folders on the wards or on posters on the walls)
- Summary algorithms or flow charts
- Integrating recommendations with care pathway documentation
- Electronic formats for website/handheld computers
- A separate guideline development document (or technical report) should be available for individuals who wish to understand how recommendations have been made and for updating recommendations later

As has been mentioned earlier in the chapter, a variety of implementation strategies needs to be used if success is to be achieved. This philosophy also holds true for the way in which the guidelines are presented. Health professionals learn in different ways and each different individual will prefer a different style. Wherever possible present the guideline in a number of different ways!

The use of interactive multi-media packages, the internet and handheld computers allows rapid and innovative ways for guidelines to be accessed, updated, and linked together. With the introduction of electronic patient records, patient symptoms and

Table 14.2

Disseminating guidelines on the web
Useful websites for disseminating guidelines
Individual College websites, e.g. RCN (www.rcn.org.uk)
National Library for Health (www.library.nhs.uk)
Stakeholder websites, e.g. patient support groups, sub-speciality interest groups
Local hospital/regional intranet sites
Create your own website (using hospital/university webspace) containing the guideline – a link from other websites to this site will cost the others nothing in terms of webspace compared to publishing the whole document

diagnoses can potentially be linked to available guidelines in relevant topics. This would allow immediate and focused dissemination of a guideline to the shop floor.

7. Dissemination – education and communication

Despite making sure you have developed rigorous evidence-based guidelines, people will still not use them if they do not know that they exist. But, even if people know they are there, if they don't understand how to use them they will just get dusty. Lack of familiarity appears to be one of the main reasons why guidelines are not used.[10]

Tips

Disseminate, disseminate, disseminate
- Pass it around the department
- Publish it in the local guideline folder
- Put it on posters in the department
- Use innovative media for publishing, e.g. mouse-mats, desk-top calendars
- Put it on the local intranet
- Put the guideline on a website (see Table 14.2)
- Involve the local opinion leaders and stakeholders to help with the above
- Spread the word, e.g. at college meetings
- Publish it in a journal
- Simplify the guideline by developing flow diagrams or care pathways
- Actively *teach* people how to implement the care pathways or flow diagrams
- Get an authoritative body to endorse it, e.g. the hospital Trust

8. Maintaining change

It is easy for people to forget their good habits quickly and fall back into bad ones again. The initial improvements brought about by the implementation of the

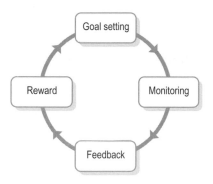

Figure 14.4 Social cognitive theory of changing/maintaining behaviour.[11]

guideline may be short lived unless a conscious effort is made to continually reinforce their use.

Reminders

Reminder mechanisms can be useful to prompt practitioners to use the guideline.[2]

- Computer decision support systems remind professionals to perform a particular action, e.g. computer records remind GPs to ask about smoking cessation during certain consultations.
- Appraisal of practitioners reminds them that demonstration of guideline use should be documented in their portfolio.
- Patients who are informed about the guideline will remind health professionals to use it.
- Care pathways provide an all-in-one solution. They allow the recommendations to be part of the patients' documentation, allowing the health professionals to write down exactly why a specific part of a guideline was not followed. The information in the documentation can then be used not only to audit practice, but also to identify areas of improvement needed (for example see Appendix 2).

Feedback

One theory of behavioural change describes the feedback mechanisms required to motivate people.[11] In fact the social cognitive theory (Figure 14.4) mimics the audit cycle in many ways.

Feedback can take a variety of forms:

- positive patient experiences;
- feedback on the success of the implementation strategies;
- results of audit.

With every guideline an ongoing audit process should be built in (see Chapter 12: The audit package). Auditing the guideline locally not only provides feedback but also reminds practitioners what the recommendations of the guideline are.

145

Longer term input

9. Evaluation of guidelines

Guideline evaluation helps to determine whether:

- there has been a change in a particular practice;
- there has been a measurable change in health outcomes.

Uptake of a guideline's recommendation also needs monitoring, so that we know whether the implementation plan has been successful or should be modified.[12] Deficiencies in the guideline can be identified through audit results and the findings used to improve and update it.

Researching the implementation of clinical guidelines

A variety of study designs can be used to evaluate whether a guideline has led to a measurable change in health outcomes. Some are more rigorous and are therefore more likely to produce less biased results. However, the study design is often limited by the ease with which it can be carried out.

Randomized trials are the most robust type of study. A randomized trial would involve one group of practitioners implementing the guideline and the other continuing with current practices. This is often difficult within one hospital or institution, because it will be very difficult to keep clinicians blinded from the development of a new guideline in the department. It may be possible to compare several hospitals, some following the guideline and others following no guideline – a cluster randomized controlled trial. This would take the co-operation of many hospitals and involve more time and resources.

Other study designs include quasi-experimental designs such as before and after studies and interrupted time series. These are weaker in design but easier to conduct. Observational or descriptive studies are not so useful at assessing outcomes but may be useful for developing an understanding of changes in behaviours of groups of clinicians.[13]

Example Box 14.1 Implementing a national evidence-based guideline locally

Guideline:
Breathing difficulty – an evidence-based guideline for the management of children presenting with acute breathing difficulty[14]

Recommendation to be implemented:
In children over the age of 2 years, without life-threatening asthma and not requiring oxygen, spacers could be used instead of nebulizers in most situations.

Strength of evidence 1, Grade of recommendation A[15]

Continued

Example Box 14.1 *Continued*

Barriers identified	Driving forces identified	Strategy used for implementation
Longstanding tradition to use nebulizers for acute asthma	Sound research evidence showing spacer devices • as good as • and having fewer side effects compared with nebulizers Also, spacers shown to • reduce admissions • and to be cheaper than nebulizers	• Papers were reviewed at the local journal club, increasing knowledge of research findings. • Nurse educators in the department were informed about performance of spacers compared to nebulizers and encouraged to disseminate knowledge to new staff. • Department managers were informed of cost–benefit of using spacers. • Audit of current practice was performed to determine admission rate following the use of nebulizers.
Experienced staff resistant to change	Consultant with respiratory interest from department identified and invited to be a stakeholder during the guideline development process	• Consultant with respiratory interest was asked to discuss the benefits of using spacers compared to nebulizers at a local meeting of senior staff, and encourage the adoption of the guideline.
Limited knowledge of existence of guideline	Regular sessions available for training staff in the department	• Member of guideline development group talked to staff about the new guideline. • Guideline was up-loaded onto hospital intranet site.
Frequently changing members of staff	Audit topics available for new staff	• Care pathway documentation was introduced with reminders of practice points written in. • Guideline use in general was promoted during induction course of new staff. • A post-implementation audit by new staff was performed. This demonstrated a decreased use of nebulizers and a decreased admission rate. Audit cycle encouraged to be repeated every year. • Positive feedback was delivered to department from managers with information regarding cost savings.

Summary

• The implementation process starts with the onset of the guideline development process.
• Use multi-faceted strategies to overcome barriers and utilize driving forces.
• Long-term input providing positive reinforcement is required to maintain changes in practice.

147

References

1. Bauchner H. Changing physician behaviour. Arch Dis Child 2001; 84:459–462.
2. NHS Centre for Reviews and Dissemination. Getting evidence into practice. Eff Health Care 1999; 5(1):1–16.

3. Prochaska J, DiClemente C. Stages and processes of self-change in smoking: towards an integrative model of change. J Consult Clin Psychol 1983; 51:390–395.

4. Rogers EM, Shoemaker FF. Communication of innovation. New York: The Free Press; 1971.

5. Grol R. Personal paper: Beliefs and evidence in changing clinical practice. BMJ 1997; 315:418–421.

6. Margolis CZ, Cretin S (eds) Implementing clinical practice guidelines. Chicago: American Hospital Association Press; 1999.

7. Department of Health. The New NHS: modern, dependable. London: The Stationery Office; 1997.

8. The Alzheimer's Society. NICE guidance on drug treatments for Alzheimer's disease. 2005 www.alzheimers.org.uk

9. Flores G et al. Pediatricians' attitudes, beliefs, and practices regarding clinical practice guidelines: a national survey. Pediatrics 2000; 105(3):496–501.

10. Mansfield C. Attitudes and behaviours towards clinical guidelines: the clinician's perspective. Qual Health Care 1995; 4:240–255.

11. Bandura A. Social foundations of thought and action: a social cognitive theory. Englewood Cliffs, NJ: Prentice Hall; 1986.

12. NHS Centre for Reviews and Dissemination. Implementing clinical practice guidelines: can guidelines be used to improve clinical practice? Effective Health Care Bulletin 1994; 8.

13. Danish Institute for Health Services Research and Development. Changing professional practice: theory and practice of clinical guidelines implementation. Copenhagen. 1999.

14. Lakhanpaul M, Armon K, Eccleston P et al. An evidence based guideline for the management of children presenting with acute breathing difficulty. 2003. Nottingham: Paediatric Accident and Emergency Research Group. www.nottingham.ac.uk/paediatric-guideline/breathingguideline.pdf

15. Cates CJ, Bara A, Crilly JA, Rowe BH. Holding chambers versus nebulisers for beta-agonist treatment of acute asthma. The Cochrane Database of Systematic Reviews 2005 Issue 1. The Cochrane Collaboration. Chichester: John Wiley.

Chapter 15

Legal issues

Richard Bowker

Aims

- To briefly describe the law in relation to clinical negligence
- To explain the legal responsibilities for the guideline user and guideline developer
- To provide tips to reduce potential litigation for guideline developers

When publishing the final guideline document, you may want to consider the legal responsibilities you have before releasing it into the public domain. Should you be contacting your legal protection scheme before proceeding? Or are you untouchable if something goes wrong when the guideline is being used by someone else?

The law and medical negligence

If a patient has suffered an adverse event, they may believe this event occurred because of negligence on behalf of their healthcare team. If a patient brings a legal action against the healthcare team then the arguments will normally be heard in a civil court. Here, the burden of proof lies with the plaintiff (the person making the allegation). The judge will make a decision for the plaintiff if *on balance of probabilities* the plaintiff's case is at least 51% probable. (In the criminal court, the jury has to believe that the prosecution's case is *beyond reasonable doubt* to find the defendant guilty.)

For the courts to accept that medical negligence did play a part, two elements must be proved. First, that the members of the healthcare team had a *duty of care* to the patient at the time, and second, the level of care provided was substandard for the patient's condition, i.e. *breaching* their duty of care.

However, negligence on its own is not enough for the patient to prove liability. It must be shown that the adverse event resulted from the negligent practice. To put it the other way round, the court must be satisfied that the adverse event would not have happened but for the negligent practice, i.e. proof of *causation*. An example can be taken from Barnet v Chelsea and Kensington Hospital Management Committee [1969] 1 QB 428. An SHO in casualty failed to examine a patient who later died from arsenic poisoning. The court did not find the defendant liable as the breach of duty did not affect the outcome – the patient would have died anyway even if a correct diagnosis had been made. Therefore, a practice may be negligent, but if causation cannot be demonstrated liability will not rest on the shoulders of the defendant.

For doctors or nurses, who look after specific patients, it is usually easy to establish whether they had a duty of care to them at the time. So let us focus on the definitions of the standard of care, noting that a guideline may be held up as such a standard.

Standard of care

The legal principles surrounding the standard of care have been established through case law. The two cases most often quoted are Bolam and Bolitho. From these cases, it is held that a health carer must act reasonably within their own ability, following practice which is respected by a responsible body of opinion and has been logically thought through.

Example Box 15.1 Bolam v Friern Hospital Management Committee [1957] 2 All ER 582

In 1954 the plaintiff, Mr Bolam, was given electroconvulsive therapy (ECT) for severe depression. The defendant, Dr Allfrey, did not use muscle relaxing drugs during the treatment and restrained Mr Bolam at the shoulders with chin support and a gag, and a pillow under his back. Mr Bolam suffered an acetabular (hip) fracture and was left with significant impairment. The counsel for the plaintiff alleged that the practice of not using muscle relaxants or not restraining Mr Bolam adequately was negligent of the defendant. The judge heard from several eminent psychiatrists, who held different views on whether the practice of not using muscle relaxants for patients undergoing ECT was a standard and acceptable practice of the day.

The judge, Mr Justice McNair, defined the standard required for acceptable practice as follows:

'A doctor is not guilty of negligence if he acted in accordance with a practice accepted as proper by a reasonable body of medical men skilled in that particular art... Putting it the other way round, a doctor is not negligent if he is acting in accordance with such a practice, merely because there is a body of opinion that takes a contrary view. At the same time, that does not mean that a medical man can obstinately and pig-headedly carry on with some old technique if it has been proved to be contrary to what is really substantially the whole of informed medical opinion.'

This has become known as the 'Bolam principle'. If a reasonable body of respectable opinion agrees with the practice, then the practice is not negligent. The courts using the Bolam principle rely on the medical profession to determine whether a practice was reasonable, by the testimonies of expert witnesses.

Example Box 15.2 Bolitho v City and Hackney Health Authority [1998] Lloyd's Rep Med 26

In 1984, Patrick Bolitho, aged two, suffered catastrophic brain damage following a respiratory then cardiac arrest in St Bartholomew's Hospital, London. He had been admitted to the hospital the night before with difficulty breathing. Dr Horn (a senior paediatric registrar, who

Continued

Example Box 15.2 *Continued*

was looking after Patrick) had been made aware by the ward's nursing staff that Patrick had suffered two sudden episodes of becoming white with acute breathing difficulties that afternoon prior to his arrest. After these brief episodes, though, he had regained full consciousness and colour, and was an active toddler again. Dr Horn did not attend to Patrick, believing that another junior doctor was attending. Tragically, a third episode of complete blockage of the respiratory system occurred, which resulted in a cardiac arrest. Patrick died some time later due to the complications of his neurological impairment.

The court found that Dr Horn had failed in her duty of care to Patrick by not reviewing him. However, the court had to decide whether the doctor, by attending him at the time requested by the nursing staff, would have made a difference to the outcome.

Expert witnesses accepted that the only way to prevent the tragic result would have been to intubate Patrick (protect his airway by inserting a tube and placing him on a breathing machine). However, the experts disagreed as to whether Patrick should have been intubated by the attending doctor on the basis of sudden respiratory distress with rapid recovery and finding a toddler running around the ward. Those experts who would not have intubated at that time helped the defendant's claim that if she had attended she would not have prevented the events which occurred.

The judge preferred the logic of the arguments put by those who would have intubated in the circumstances. However, the judge also held that, although the views of the expert witnesses were diametrically opposed, both represented a responsible body of professional opinion supported by distinguished and truthful experts. The judge refused to substitute his own lay views for those of the medical experts. Therefore, the judge held that, if Dr Horn had attended and not intubated, she would have reached the standard of care required. Accordingly, he held that it had not been proved that the admitted breach of duty by the defendant had caused the catastrophe.

Dr Horn was found not guilty of negligence. The case went to appeal on the basis that the judge had wrongly treated the *Bolam* test as requiring him to accept the views of one truthful body of expert professional advice, even though he was not persuaded by its logical force.

The judgment of the appeal courts was summarized by Lord Browne-Wilkinson:

'...in my view, the court is not bound to hold that a defendant doctor escapes liability for negligent treatment or diagnosis just because he leads evidence from a number of medical experts who are genuinely of opinion that the defendant's treatment or diagnosis accorded with sound medical practice ... the court has to be satisfied that the exponents of the body of opinion relied upon can demonstrate that such opinion has a logical basis. In particular in cases involving, as they often do, the weighing of risks against benefits, the judge before accepting a body of opinion as being responsible, reasonable or respectable, will need to be satisfied that, in forming their views, the experts have directed their minds to the question of comparative risks and benefits and have reached a defensible conclusion on the matter.'

The appeal court judged that the defendant was not liable, as the expert witnesses had all provided a logical basis for their respected opinions.

This ruling has been termed the 'Bolitho gloss on Bolam'. It means that, rather than naively relying on the opinions of medical experts, the court must be satisfied that the opinion is logical, and that the risks and benefits have been reasonably balanced in the eyes of the court, not just the experts.

Applying the law to guidelines

Guideline users

Following a guideline

If a guideline is followed the courts will want that guidance to satisfy the Bolam and Bolitho principles, i.e. that the guideline is reasonable, logical and respected by a competent body of medical opinion. These issues have precedents in case law and can be demonstrated by the Bland and Early cases.

Example Box 15.3 The Tony Bland case (Airedale Trust v Bland [1993] 4 Med LR 39)

This widely reported case involved withdrawal of medical treatment from a young man who was in a persistent vegetative state (PVS). British Medical Association (BMA) guidelines on PVS were referred to and supported by judges in the case. Lord Goff stated:

'Study of this document left me in no doubt that, if a doctor treating a PVS patient acts in accordance with the medical practice now being evolved by the Medical Ethics Committee of the BMA, he will be acting with the benefit of guidance from a responsible and competent body of relevant professional opinion.'

Example Box 15.4 The Early case (Early v Newham Health Authority [1994] 5 Med LR 214)

This case concerned an unsuccessful intubation and the alleged incompetence of an anaesthetist. Hospital guidance on failed intubation was a central feature of the case. It was alleged that the guidance was faulty. The procedure for failed intubation was as follows:

'Where the intubation fails, cricoid pressure should be maintained, ventilate with oxygen, do not give a second dose of suxamethonium, do not persist with repeated attempts at intubation, turn the patient on side, call for help. If the procedure is not for a life-threatening condition, continue oxygenation, allow the patient to wake up.'

The court looked at the procedure development process and the degree to which the procedure was generally accepted in the medical community. It was established that it had been put before the division of anaesthesia in the hospital and that the consultants had decided that this was the proper procedure to follow. Minutes of this discussion had been kept.

Deputy Judge Benett stated, *'I am quite satisfied ... that I am dealing with a competent medical authority who had applied its mind to this problem and came up with a reasonable solution.'*

No negligence was found in the end as the anaesthetist had followed a guideline which was sound.

For the guideline user, some knowledge of the processes and checks the guideline has undergone during its development is useful. It would be impossible and impractical for everyone to perform an AGREE appraisal on every guideline they were about to use. They should therefore ask the following questions:

- Has it been approved, and therefore appraised, by the local guideline committee?
- Has it been endorsed externally, e.g. by a Royal College?
- Is there a review date to ensure the guidance is contemporary?
- Does it make sense and seem reasonable for this patient?

Not following a guideline

Is a practitioner automatically found guilty of negligence if there is a guideline available but it is not used in a particular case? The answer is 'no, not automatically', but it will depend on the practice used in each individual case. Can the decisions that were made in the case stand up to the Bolam and Bolitho principles? What were the specific characteristics of this case that led to a divergence from a guideline? Is there a body of respected opinion which agrees that deviation from the guideline was both reasonable and logical?

Professional judgement is never superseded by a guideline.[1] Guidelines are tools to help professionals make judgements. They should not be seen as an excuse for the practitioner to run on auto-pilot. Blindly following a guideline irrespective of the needs of the individual patient would be seen as negligent in the eyes of the court.

Example Box 15.5 Penney, Palmer and Cannon v East Kent HA [2000] Lloyd's Rep Mod 11

This case concerned cervical smear tests and negligence allegations concerning interpretation of findings. Some slides had been labelled 'negative' when they showed slight abnormalities. No medical follow-up was arranged for the claimants, who went on to develop cancer of the cervix. The standards of the Cervical Screening Programme (CSP) were cited and were not complied with in this case. Consequently the health authority was found negligent.

At the appeal, it was argued that the Bolam test should have been applied to the cervical smear slide results, as different experts had stated that the results could be interpreted in a number of ways. The trial judge had not used the Bolam test and had instead relied on a test of screener satisfaction, known as the 'absolute confidence' test, which was incorporated into the clinical guidelines of the CSP, which all the experts seemed to endorse. The trial judge had used this test in deciding the issue of the correct standard of care and whether this had been met.

It was accepted that the national cervical screening programme could not identify all abnormal smear tests. However, a judge was entitled to conclude that a test contained obvious abnormalities even though there was conflicting expert evidence on that issue. On the judge's findings, the screeners should at least have concluded that the slides were difficult to interpret and therefore the slides should have failed the absolute confidence test. The screeners did not follow the guidance of the CSP by referring the samples for further investigation and therefore acted negligently.

The courts may use a particular guideline as evidence of a standard of care expected in certain situations (see the Penney case above), but this is just one of many sources of evidence.[2] The courts recognize the importance of clinicians exercising clinical discretion. It is useful for the courts to understand the decision-making processes in each case by clearly documenting the reasoning behind judgements at the time they are made.

If a practitioner is deviating from a guideline they normally use, they should ask themselves the following:

- Can I justify these decisions for this patient?
- Is it clear in the records why these decisions are justified?

Guideline developers

Legal responsibility in guideline development

The development of a clinical guideline should lead to a practice which is respected by a responsible body of opinion and has been logically thought through. Well produced guidelines therefore should be at no risk of liability.

In the UK, there have been no cases which have found a practice guideline to be the cause of an adverse event. Therefore, currently there are no precedent cases to hold up as examples of when a guideline development group might be held responsible for patient care. The Department of Health has commented, 'It would be difficult to establish that a duty of care is owed to the patient by the college or professional body issuing the guidelines.[3]

However, others have argued that it is possible that liability in negligence might be imposed upon those who publish clinical guidelines.[4] If the guideline development group (GDG) made recommendations leading to a particular medical procedure being adopted, which they could foresee would cause more harm than good to the patients, then they may be held liable.

154

Tips

Reducing potential litigation in guideline development
Use the AGREE Instrument to help during the development process
Document the guideline development process
Be transparent about the decision-making process
Ensure the guideline is appraised before publication
Incorporate a review date into the guideline

The Department of Health has given legal advice for guideline developers,[3] which fits entirely with the AGREE Instrument.[5] The law does not allow inexperience as an excuse for negligence (see the Wilsher case below). Therefore, ensure that the guideline clearly states who should be using the guideline and to whom the guideline should apply.

Example Box 15.6 Wilsher v Essex Area Health Authority [1988] 1 All ER 871

A premature infant had an umbilical arterial catheter inserted to monitor the oxygen in the infant's blood. Unfortunately the catheter was inserted incorrectly into the umbilical vein by a junior doctor on duty. This mistake was not spotted on X-ray by either this doctor or his supervising registrar. Because of this error extra oxygen was given to the baby, who went on to develop retinopathy of prematurity, known to be related to excess oxygen delivery. The infant was subsequently blind.

Continued

Example Box 15.6 *Continued*

The case went via the Court of Appeal to the House of Lords on the point of causation. However, the Appeal Court clarified the test for standard of care for a trainee. This is not related to the experience of the individual trainee, but the standard expected of a person who fills the post that doctor is employed in and the tasks elected to be performed by that person. A junior registrar in a senior registrar's post may therefore be judged according to the standards of a senior registrar.

By applying this test individually to the doctors in this case, both would have been found to be in breach of duty of care. The Court of Appeal did, however, accept that by seeking advice from a senior the trainee doctor satisfied the necessary standard of care required when exercising a specialist skill. The Court of Appeal held the more senior doctor to be negligent, as he should have spotted the error of his junior.

Lord Justice Glidewell said: *'In my view, the law requires the trainee or learner to be judged by the same standard as his more experienced colleagues. If it did not, inexperience would frequently be urged as a defence to an action for professional negligence.'*

The importance of building a review date into guidelines has been highlighted by the Department of Health[3] and the AGREE Instrument.[5] Patients expect, as the courts do, practitioners to keep their practice up to date. By incorporating a review date into the guideline, the user can be confident that the advice is or is not contemporary.

Example Box 15.7 Crawford v Board of Governors of Charing Cross Hospital, The Times, 8 December, 1953

The plaintiff developed a brachial palsy (nerve damage to the arm) after his arm had been positioned at an angle of 80° to his body during surgery. Six months prior to the operation, an article in the *Lancet* had pointed out the danger of brachial palsy when the arm was kept in such an extended position. The anaesthetist had not read the article in question and the judge, at first instance, held the defendant liable for negligence.

The Court of Appeal overturned the ruling and found the anaesthetist not negligent. Lord Denning stated, *'...it would, I think, be putting too high a burden on a medical man to say that he has to read every article appearing in the current medical press; and it would be quite wrong to suggest that a medical man is negligent because he does not at once put into operation the suggestions which some contributor or other might make in a medical journal. The time may come in a particular case when a new recommendation may be so well proved and so well known, and so well accepted that it should be adopted, but that was not so in this case'.*

Therefore, guideline developers do not need to be contacting their legal protection scheme, so long as they have developed and documented carefully the guideline they are about to publish.

Summary

- Guidelines must be reasonable, logical and up to date.
- Document the decisions taken when developing or using guidelines.
- External appraisal demonstrates the recommendations are respected by a responsible body of opinion.

References

1. Tingle J. Do guidelines have legal implications? Arch Dis Child 2002; 86:387–388.
2. Hirshfield E. Use of practice parameters as standards of care and in health care reform: a view from the American Medical Association. J Qual Improvement 1993; 19:322–329.
3. Department of Health. Clinical guidelines: using clinical guidelines to improve patient care within the NHS. London: DOH; 1996.
4. Stern K. Clinical guidelines and negligence; In: Deighan M, Hitch S, eds. Clinical effectiveness liability: from guidelines to cost-effective practice. Brentwood: Earlybrave Publications; 1995, p 127–135.
5. The AGREE Collaboration. Appraisal of guidelines for research and evaluation (AGREE Instrument). 2001. www.agreecollaboration.org

The AGREE Appraisal Instrument

Reprinted with kind permission from The AGREE Collaboration. Appraisal of Guidelines for Research and Evaluation (AGREE) Instrument © St George's Hospital Medical School, London, June 2001. Reprinted with amendments September 2001.

The following is adapted to provide the guideline developer with insight into how the guideline will be appraised. To use the assessment tool for appraisal, visit www. agreecollaboration.org for instructions and the full version.

Purpose of the AGREE Instrument.

The purpose of the Appraisal of Guidelines Research & Evaluation (AGREE) Instrument is to provide a framework for assessing the quality of clinical practice guidelines.

Clinical practice guidelines are 'systematically developed statements to assist practitioner and patient decisions about appropriate health care for specific clinical circumstances'[1]. Their purpose is 'to make explicit recommendations with a definite intent to influence what clinicians do'[2].

By quality of clinical practice guidelines we mean the confidence that the potential biases of guideline development have been addressed adequately and that the recommendations are both internally and externally valid, and are feasible for practice. This process involves taking into account the benefits, harms and costs of the recommendations, as well as the practical issues attached to them. Therefore, the assessment includes judgements about the methods used for developing the guidelines, the content of the final recommendations, and the factors linked to their uptake.

The AGREE Instrument assesses both the quality of the reporting, and the quality of some aspects of recommendations. It provides an assessment of the predicted validity of a guideline, that is the likelihood that it will achieve its intended outcome. It does not assess the impact of a guideline on patients' outcomes.

Most of the criteria contained in the AGREE Instrument are based on theoretical assumptions rather than on empirical evidence. They have been developed through discussions between researchers from several countries who have extensive experience and knowledge of clinical guidelines. Thus, the AGREE Instrument should be perceived as reflecting the current state of knowledge in the field.

Assessment criteria and user guides

SCOPE AND PURPOSE

1. The overall objective(s) of the guideline is(are) specifically described.

| Strongly Agree | 4 | 3 | 2 | 1 | Strongly Disagree |

This deals with the potential health impact of a guideline on society and populations of patients.

The overall objective(s) of the guideline should be described in detail and the expected health benefits from the guideline should be specific to the clinical problem. For example specific statements would be:
- Preventing (long term) complications of patients with diabetes mellitus;
- Lowering the risk of subsequent vascular events in patients with previous myocardial infarction;
- Rational prescribing of antidepressants in a cost-effective way.

2. The clinical question(s) covered by the guideline is(are) specifically described.

| Strongly Agree | 4 | 3 | 2 | 1 | Strongly Disagree |

A detailed description of the clinical questions covered by the guideline should be provided, particularly for the key recommendations (see item 17). Following the examples provided in question 1:
- How many times a year should the HbA1c be measured in patients with diabetes mellitus?
- What should the daily aspirin dosage for patients with proven acute myocardial infarction be?
- Are selective serotonin reuptake inhibitors (SSRIs) more cost-effective than tricyclic antidepressants (TCAs) in treatment of patients with depression?

3. The patients to whom the guideline is meant to apply are specifically described.

| Strongly Agree | 4 | 3 | 2 | 1 | Strongly Disagree |

There should be a clear description of the target population to be covered by a guideline. The age range, sex, clinical description, comorbidity may be provided. For example:
- A guideline on the management of diabetes mellitus only includes patients with non-insulin dependent diabetes mellitus and excludes patients with cardiovascular comorbidity.
- A guideline on the management of depression only includes patients with major depression, according to the DSM-IV criteria, and excludes patients with psychotic symptoms and children.
- A guideline on screening of breast cancer only includes women, aged between 50 and 70 years, with no history of cancer and with no family history of breast cancer.

STAKEHOLDER INVOLVEMENT

4. The guideline development group includes individuals from all the relevant professional groups.

Strongly Agree | 4 | 3 | 2 | 1 | Strongly Disagree

This item refers to the professionals who were involved at some stage of the development process. This may include members of the steering group, the research team involved in selecting and reviewing/rating the evidence and individuals involved in formulating the final recommendations. This item excludes individuals who have externally reviewed the guideline (see Item 13). Information about the composition, discipline and relevant expertise of the guideline development group should be provided.

5. The patients' views and preferences have been sought.

Strongly Agree | 4 | 3 | 2 | 1 | Strongly Disagree

Information about patients' experiences and expectations of health care should inform the development of clinical guidelines. There are various methods for ensuring that patients' perspectives inform guideline development. For example, the development group could involve patients' representatives, information could be obtained from patient interviews, literature reviews of patients' experiences could be considered by the group. There should be evidence that this process has taken place.

6. The target users of the guideline are clearly defined.

Strongly Agree | 4 | 3 | 2 | 1 | Strongly Disagree

The target users should be clearly defined in the guideline, so they can immediately determine if the guideline is relevant to them. For example, the target users for a guideline on low back pain may include general practitioners, neurologists, orthopaedic surgeons, rheumatologists and physiotherapists.

7. The guideline has been piloted among target users.

Strongly Agree | 4 | 3 | 2 | 1 | Strongly Disagree

A guideline should have been pre-tested for further validation amongst its intended end users prior to publication. For example, a guideline may have been piloted in one or several primary care practices or hospitals. This process should be documented.

RIGOUR OF DEVELOPMENT

8. Systematic methods were used to search for evidence.

Strongly Agree | 4 | 3 | 2 | 1 | Strongly Disagree

Details of the strategy used to search for evidence should be provided including search terms used, sources consulted and dates of the literature covered. Sources may include electronic databases (e.g. MEDLINE, EMBASE, CINAHL), databases of systematic reviews (e.g. the Cochrane Library, DARE), handsearching journals, reviewing conference proceedings and other guidelines (e.g. the US National Guideline Clearinghouse, the German Guidelines Clearinghouse).

9. The criteria for selecting the evidence are clearly described.

Strongly Agree | 4 | 3 | 2 | 1 | Strongly Disagree

Criteria for including/excluding evidence identified by the search should be provided. These criteria should be explicitly described and reasons for including and excluding evidence should be clearly stated. For example, guideline authors may decide to only include evidence from randomised clinical trials and to exclude articles not written in English.

10. The methods used for formulating the recommendations are clearly described.

Strongly Agree | 4 | 3 | 2 | 1 | Strongly Disagree

There should be a description of the methods used to formulate the recommendations and how final decisions were arrived at. Methods include for example, a voting system, formal consensus techniques (e.g. Delphi, Glaser techniques). Areas of disagreement and methods of resolving them should be specified.

11. The health benefits, side effects and risks have been considered in formulating the recommendations.

Strongly Agree | 4 | 3 | 2 | 1 | Strongly Disagree

The guideline should consider health benefits, side effects, and risks of the recommendations. For example, a guideline on the management of breast cancer may include a discussion on the overall effects on various final outcomes. These may include: survival, quality of life, adverse effects, and symptom management or a discussion comparing one treatment option to another. There should be evidence that these issues have been addressed.

RIGOUR OF DEVELOPMENT

12. There is an explicit link between the recommendations and the supporting evidence.

Strongly Agree | 4 | 3 | 2 | 1 | Strongly Disagree

There should be an explicit link between the recommendations and the evidence on which they are based. Each recommendation should be linked with a list of references on which it is based.

13. The guideline has been externally reviewed by experts prior to its publication.

Strongly Agree | 4 | 3 | 2 | 1 | Strongly Disagree

A guideline should be reviewed externally before it is published. Reviewers should not have been involved in the development group and should include some experts in the clinical area and some methodological experts. Patients' representatives may also be included. A description of the methodology used to conduct the external review should be presented, which may include a list of the reviewers and their affiliation.

14. A procedure for updating the guideline is provided.

Strongly Agree | 4 | 3 | 2 | 1 | Strongly Disagree

Guidelines need to reflect current research. There should be a clear statement about the procedure for updating the guideline. For example, a timescale has been given, or a standing panel receives regularly updated literature searches and makes changes as required.

CLARITY AND PRESENTATION

15. The recommendations are specific and unambiguous.

Strongly Agree | 4 | 3 | 2 | 1 | Strongly Disagree

A recommendation should provide a concrete and precise description of which management is appropriate in which situation and in what patient group, as permitted by the body of evidence.
- An example of a specific recommendation is: Antibiotics have to be prescribed in children of two years or older with acute otitis media if the complaint last longer than three days or if the complaint increase after the consultation despite adequate treatment with painkillers; in these cases amoxycillin should be given for 7 days (supplied with a dosage scheme).
- An example of a vague recommendation is: Antibiotics are indicated for cases with an abnormal or complicated course.
However, evidence is not always clear cut and there may be uncertainty about the best management. In this case the uncertainty should be stated in the guideline.

16. The different options for management of the condition are clearly presented.

Strongly Agree | 4 | 3 | 2 | 1 | Strongly Disagree

162

A guideline should consider the different possible options for screening, prevention, diagnosis or treatment of the condition it covers. These possible options should be clearly presented in the guideline. For example, a recommendation on the management of depression may contain the following alternatives:
a. Treatment with TCA
b. Treatment with SSRI
c. Psychotherapy
d. Combination of pharmacological and psychological therapy

17. Key recommendations are easily identifiable.

| Strongly Agree | 4 | 3 | 2 | 1 | Strongly Disagree |

Users should be able to find the most relevant recommendations easily. These recommendations answer the main clinical questions that have been covered by the guideline. They can be identified in different ways. For example, they can be summarised in a box, typed in bold, underlined or presented as flow charts or algorithms.

18. The guideline is supported with tools for application.

| Strongly Agree | 4 | 3 | 2 | 1 | Strongly Disagree |

For a guideline to be effective it needs to be disseminated and implemented with additional materials. These may include for example, a summary document, or a quick reference guide, educational tools, patients' leaflets, computer support, and should be provided with the guideline.

APPLICABILITY

19. The potential organisational barriers in applying the recommendations have been discussed.

| Strongly Agree | 4 | 3 | 2 | 1 | Strongly Disagree |

163

Applying the recommendations may require changes in the current organisation of care within a service or a clinic which may be a barrier to using them in daily practice. Organisational changes that may be needed in order to apply the recommendations should be discussed. For example:
i. A guideline on stroke may recommend that care should be co-ordinated through stroke units and stroke services.
ii. A guideline on diabetes in primary care may require that patients are seen and followed up in diabetic clinics.

20. The potential cost implications of applying the recommendations have been considered.

| Strongly Agree | 4 | 3 | 2 | 1 | Strongly Disagree |

The recommendations may require additional resources in order to be applied. For example, there may be a need for more specialised staff, new equipment, expensive drug treatment. These may have cost implications for health care budgets. There should be a discussion of the potential impact on resources in the guideline.

21. The guideline presents key review criteria for monitoring and/or audit purposes.

| Strongly Agree | 4 | 3 | 2 | 1 | Strongly Disagree |

Measuring the adherence to a guideline can enhance its use. This requires clearly defined review criteria that are derived from the key recommendations in the guideline. These should be presented. Examples of review criteria are:
- The HbA1c should be <8.0%.
- The level of diastolic blood pressure should be <95 mmHg.
- If complaints of acute otitis media lasts longer than three days amoxicillin should be prescribed.

EDITORIAL INDEPENDENCE

22. The guideline is editorially independent from the funding body.

| Strongly Agree | 4 | 3 | 2 | 1 | Strongly Disagree |

Some guidelines are developed with external funding (e.g. Government funding, charity organisations, pharmaceutical companies). Support may be in the form of financial contribution for the whole development, or for parts of it, e.g. printing of the guidelines. There should be an explicit statement that the views or interests of the funding body have not influenced the final recommendations. Please note: If it is stated that a guideline was developed without external funding, then you should answer 'Strongly Agree'.

23. Conflicts of interest of guideline development members have been recorded.

| Strongly Agree | 4 | 3 | 2 | 1 | Strongly Disagree |

There are circumstances when members of the development group may have conflicts of interest. For example, this would apply to a member of the development group whose research on the topic covered by the guideline is also funded by a pharmaceutical company. There should be an explicit statement that all group members have declared whether they have any conflict of interest.

Appendix 2

Care pathways

An integrated care pathway (ICP) is a multidisciplinary outline of anticipated care, placed in an appropriate timeframe, to help a patient with a specific condition or set of symptoms to move progressively through a clinical experience to positive outcomes.[1] ICPs can be used as a tool to incorporate local and national guidelines into everyday practice, manage clinical risk and meet the requirements of clinical governance.

A care pathway can be viewed as an extension of a clinical guideline, helping to organize and assess the implementation of the recommendations.

To illustrate the value of using a pathway of care let's look at an example from industry. There is more than one way of assembling a car, but a manufacturing *pathway* will describe one way of assembling one car on a production line. This is the best and most efficient way of delivering a product which the customer wants. If everyone was trying to do things in their own way within the same organization, then there would be obvious variation in the quality of the output.[1] Patients should not be viewed as commodities but the process of care can be standardized, and a care pathway is one way of implementing standardization.

Care pathways are often specific to a patient population or diagnosis, e.g. deep vein thrombosis or paediatric breathing difficulties. They are often the only source of documentation for that patient episode and are used by all professionals.

In the example below, 'Suspected deep vein thrombosis care pathway' (permission to adapt kindly provided by Glenis Hawkins, Integrated Care Pathway & Modernisation Team, Royal Berkshire and Battle Hospitals NHS Trust), nurse, doctor and radiological assessments are all written on the one document. All the recommendations of the hospital's guideline are present in the document. The process of the patient journey with a deep vein thrombosis is clearly organized to reduce delay and improve patient satisfaction as well as outcome. (Please note that, in the example below, the entire pathway has not been reproduced but just the first few pages.)

Further examples of care pathways and how to develop them can be found at the National Library for Health (www.library.nhs.uk/pathways). With the advent of electronic patient records, care pathways are likely to become integrated into hospital admissions and GP episodes more and more.

Reference

1. Anonymous. On care pathways. Bondolier Forum. 2003 (July). www.jr2.ox.ac.uk/bandolier/Extraforbando/Forum2.pdf

DVT Unit

Suspected Deep Vein Thrombosis (DVT)
Care Pathway

Patients Name....................
NHS no.
(Affix patient label)
Time of arrival................hrs

Patient likes to be known as

Baseline observations

BP	Pulse	Temperature	O$_2$ saturation
Pain score	**Weight**	**Other**	
Allergies			

	Initial	Reason for variance and action taken
Baseline observations within normal limits for patient		
Pain score of <5 or acceptable to patient		
Demographics obtained		
Explanation of DVT assessment/ procedure given to patient		
Essential bloods taken **Blood card marked with urgent sticker** D-dimer ☐ time....... Coag screen ☐ FBC ☐ IPA ☐		

Presenting complaint

History of presenting complaint

Chest pain Y ☐ N ☐   Dyspnoea Y ☐ N ☐   Haemoptysis Y ☐ N ☐

If yes to any of the above patient must be reviewed by a doctor (page 10)

Additional risk factors for deep vein thrombosis (tick relevant box(es))

COC/HRT	☐	Family history of DVT or PE	☐
Obesity	☐	Recent long haul travel	☐

Current medication							
Name	Dose	Frequency	Route	Name	Dose	Frequency	Route

Limb examination

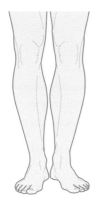 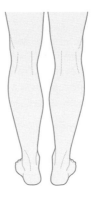

DVT pretest probability score (modified from Wells P, Anderson D. Lancet 1997; 350:1795) *(if present, place tick in box(es))*		
	Tick	**Score**
Active cancer (treatment within previous 6 months or current palliative treatment)		1
Paralysis, paresis or recent plaster immobilisation of lower extremities		1
Recently bedridden 3 or more days or major surgery within previous 12 weeks		1
Localised tenderness along veins		1
Entire leg swollen		1
Calf swelling >3 cm than asymptomatic leg (10 cm below tibial tuberosity) Symptomatic leg........cm Asymptomatic leg......cm **Difference**.........		1
Pitting oedema confined to symptomatic leg		1
Collateral superficial veins (non varicose)		1
Previously documented deep vein thrombosis/PE		1
Alternative diagnosis is likely or greater than of a DVT		−2
Pregnant Y ☐ N ☐ Six weeks post partum/miscarriage Y ☐ N ☐		2
Completed by............................		
Score Low 0 ☐ Moderate 1–2 ☐ High 3+ ☐		
D-dimer result .... (<130 = negative) **Time**.................		

Blood results

Hb		WBC		Platelets	
INR		APTR		Other	
Na	K+		Urea		Creatinine

Name   DOB   Date

Management plan

☐   Blood results reviewed.
      Within expected range   (exclude D-dimer)   Y ☐   N ☐
      If no, abnormal results discussed with Dr   ☐   Outcome documented on page 9

☐   Low/moderate probability & D-dimer <130 **excludes DVT.**
☐   Low/moderate probability & D-dimer >130 **requires ultrasound/venogram**
☐   High probability (regardless of D-dimer) **requires ultrasound/venogram**
Note, Registrar or Consultant to review patient if management plan is to be varianced.   Signed............................

DVT excluded	Initial	Reason for variance and action taken
Results and information given to patient and carer		
No additional relevant clinical symptoms. If yes refer to medical team		
Patient fit for discharge ***Note all patients with active cancer must be reviewed by medical/oncology team***		
Patient asked to return to GP		
Discharge letter sent to GP		
Date and time of discharge **Discharged by**		

Possible DVT		Initial	Reason for variance and action taken
Need for venogram/ultrasound explained to patient			
Pre venogram check list	Yes	No	Record additional information
If patient is pregnant, Ionising Radiation form completed & sent to Xray with ICP			
Previous reaction to contrast media?			
Patient on Metformin (if yes, patient told to withhold drug for 48 hours after venogram)			
Patient aware to return to Radiology following day at.................for venogram			
Stat dose of Tinzaparin given for moderate/high probability score & positive D-dimer **excluding** patients with active cancer who should be seen by medical/oncology team ***(low probability and positive D-dimer doesn't require Tinzaparin overnight)***			
Patient discharged home with interim letter			
Care pathway taken to radiology department for 9am the following morning			

Ultrasound/venogram request on next page

Name   DOB   Date

Ultrasound/venogram request
Side Left ☐   Right ☐
Signature of nurse requesting venogram...................... Bleep no............

Ultrasound ☐ / **venogram** ☐ **report**		
Date	**Time**	

Ultrasound solidus Venogram result:
Negative ☐
Positive ☐   Above knee ☐ Iliac vein involvement Y ☐ N ☐
                Below knee ☐
If limited ultrasound performed (not a full leg) and a high probability, a repeat ultrasound booked for 7–10 days ☐ Date booked .../.../...
                Signature of Radiologist/Radiographer................................

Following venogram/ultrasound, patient to return to DVT assessment unit

Information giving	Initial	Reason for variance and action taken
Results & information given to patient & carer		
For patients that have had a limited ultrasound and have a high probability only Patient aware to return to Radiology for a repeat ultrasound on ....../....../..... at ....../...... hrs		
Patient discharged home with interim letter		

Please note, patient doesn't require Tinzaparin cover   See protocol page 2

Date and time of discharge	Discharged by

DVT excluded by full leg ultrasound/ venogram or limited ultrasound with low/moderate probability	Initial	Reason for variance and action taken
No additional relevant clinical symptoms. If yes refer to medical team		
Patient fit for discharge *Note all patients with active cancer must be reviewed by medical/oncology team*		
Patient asked to return to GP		
Discharge letter sent to GP		
Date and time of discharge	Discharged by nurse...............................	

Confirmed DVT

Suitability for outpatient treatment

Medical criteria	Initial	Reason for variance and action taken
No signs of breathlessness		
No clinical evidence of an iliac vein thrombosis		
No clinical evidence of active bleeding		
No active peptic ulceration (diagnosed within previous 4 weeks)		
No familial/acquired bleeding disorder		
Active cancer patients only. Medical/oncology team have agreed to outpatient treatment		
Cautionary criteria		
No history of a specific thrombophilic disorder		
No past history of heparin induced thrombocytopenia		
Patient is not pregnant		
Normal coagulation screen and normal platelet count		
If any of above statements have been varianced, refer to SHO *Patients with suspected or confirmed PE (as well as DVT) may be suitable for domiciliary protocol, but must be included in clinical trial until safety established*		
Patient education		
Patient informed of rationale upon which outpatient treatment is based		
Options of self administration or community nurse based care discussed		
Social criteria		
Patient/carer able to comprehend home care package		
Patient/carer has access to telephone		
Patient mobility does not affect their normal activities		
Administration		
Patient to self administer Patient confident and competent on LMW Heparin dose and is capable of self administration **Community care to administer** GP's surgery/community nurse phoned prior to discharge **Hospital to administer** Patient to attend Victoria ward/DVT unit		
Suitable for outpatient treatment		
Patient suitable for outpatient treatment		**If no, patient to be admitted to ward** ....
Tinzaparin prescribed (page 12) for patients returning to hospital for injections		
Outpatient appointments made: Consultant physician (6 weeks) ☐ AC clinic referral completed and sent ☐ **AC clinic faxed yellow discharge letter** ☐		
DVT Discharge letter completed (refer to pages 12,13 for dosing & duration schedule)		

Index

Notes
Page numbers in *italics* refer to boxed material, figures and tables.

175